Assessing older people

A practical guide for health professionals

Assessing older people

A practical guide for health professionals

Susan Koch

Senior Lecturer, School of Nursing, La Trobe University, Melbourne

Sally Garratt

Associate Professor, School of Nursing, La Trobe University,
Melbourne and
Head, Nursing Education & Clinical Support Unit, Caulfield General
Medical Centre, Melbourne
(Formerly Director of Nursing, Elanora, Vision Australia Foundation,
Melbourne)

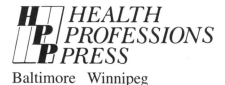
HEALTH
PROFESSIONS
PRESS
Baltimore Winnipeg

Health Professions Press, Inc.
PO Box 10624
Baltimore, MD 21285-0624
U.S.A
www.healthpropress.com

© 2001 Elsevier Australia
A division of Reed International Books Australia (Pty) Ltd
ABN 70 001 002 357

ISBN 1-932529-00-4

Cover design by Pamela Horsnell, Juno Creative Services
Printed and bound in Australia by Ligare

dedication

To all those with a passion for providing the best care possible to older people

contents

foreword

Caring for older people has traditionally been seen as boring, lacking challenge, requiring few skills and little knowledge, and being less attractive to 'good' nurses. One reason for this of course is the pervasive ageism that devalues older people and their care. However, there has been another reason and that is that many nurses who did work with older people provided little more than custody and thus confirmed the stereotype, creating a vicious circle. Where staff believe they can do nothing and the older person is simply at the 'end of the line', it can be demoralising and job dissatisfaction will ensure high staff turnover, increased sick leave and problems recruiting and retaining well qualified staff. Such a depressing environment can encourage nurses to distance themselves by depersonalising the older person and denying their basic human rights.

Changes in the broader society have supported the view, long held by skilled gerontic nurses, that custody is a totally inappropriate model for aged care. It is never the case that 'nothing can be done'. While ever there is life, people have goals; when cognitive decline or other illness and disability prevent the person from communicating their goals it cannot be assumed they have none. On the contrary, it becomes vital that the nurse seeks as much information as possible about the person and their life choices so that they can anticipate what the person would have wanted and how they might display consent, pleasure or unhappiness in relation to any decisions the nurses (or others) make in relation to their care.

There is now a plethora of evidence to demonstrate that holistic care—tailored to the individual—produces positive health outcomes. There is also evidence to show that nurses have greater job satisfaction in situations where they feel able to influence care decisions and see that through their interventions quality of life is increased. If the recognition of the individual in context requires further encouragement, the general societal trends towards greater individual choice and the litigation that increasingly follows unsubstantiated unilateral care decisions, provide it. Where then might nurses start if they are to provide contemporary, high quality care? The obvious place is with assessment. Comprehensive and specific, focused assessments provide the data which can then inform care practices and direct the nurse toward research that may be needed to assist the person to draw upon and meet their own goals. Identifying the gaps alerts the nurse to where care should be directed. Such an approach also reduces the likelihood that nurses will foster dependency by doing for the older person what they are capable of doing for themselves. Concentrating on goals and strengths creates a positive environment, which facilitates a sense of worth.

Susan Koch and Sally Garratt have brought together a team of experts who provide the rationale and the tools to assist nurses to understand the 'whys and hows' of assessing older people. This is an excellent text that is informative, practical and, most importantly for me, passionate about the humanity and personhood of the older person. When nurses recognise the possibilities and experience the satisfaction that flow from good assessment, the ageist belief that 'nothing can be done' will be replaced by an optimistic realisation that there is much that can be done. Nurses who read this book will be well placed to deliver high quality health care for older people. I commend the editors and authors for managing to deliver a rigorous and yet accessible text that values and centres older people.

Rhonda Nay

Professor of Gerontic Nursing
La Trobe University, Melbourne

preface

This book is a guide to assist health care professionals with the development of their assessment skills. The book provides primarily nurses with comprehensive information related to holistic assessment of the older person and draws upon research-based evidence related to normal and abnormal changes associated with ageing. Assessment of older people requires a practitioner to gather data, make sense of the information, and make informed decisions from the data that will lead to effective planning of care strategies. Although the assessment process is always undertaken within a current social and political framework, we have chosen not to explore this as other texts have already done so; for example, *Nursing Older People: Issues and Innovations* (Nay, R. and Garratt, S. 1999, MacLennan & Petty, Sydney).

The skill development required for professional assessment does not change, regardless of the sociopolitical climate; however, thorough professional assessment will always be essential for the provision of quality care. This text has been arranged to guide the reader through study questions that will facilitate self-directed learning. Assessment tools have been included to illustrate how the process can be recorded; however, these are examples only and the reader must bear in mind that adaptation to specific environments is often necessary. All case studies and examples in this book employ pseudonyms and details have been altered to protect privacy.

part 1 the foundation for assessment

Part 1 of the book examines the decision-making process, holistic assessment and the cultural context that underpins the assessment process. The concepts and principles discussed in these chapters will be found to underpin the remainder of the book. While Chapter 1 illustrates an eight-step problem solving approach, readers must recognise that this model does not mean that all care issues are problems but rather that it should reflect the *thinking process* of the assessor. A systematic process assists in identifying major issues of immediate concern, and provides knowledge of the person and their world in a manageable format. This task would otherwise be overwhelmingly complex.

part 2 assessment for clinical practice

Part 2 of the book examines the assessment process in more detail. These chapters provide the reader with examples of assessment tools useful for the gathering of specific data. The reader will be exposed to various clinical practice issues and offered guidelines and protocols to develop their assessment skills. The issues outlined have environmental and social ramifications and are broader than physical body systems.

acknowledgments

A number of people have assisted in the development of this book. We wish to thank Sue Hee and Catherine Watts for their tireless administrative assistance in preparation of the manuscript. They had the unenviable task of making the layout of the chapters consistent, ensuring references were correctly written and cited, and formatting disks from a wide variety of programs to the end product you have before you. Professor Rhonda Nay has been an influential supporter and colleague throughout the project. Our publishers, MacLennan & Petty, deserve special mention for their patience and support during the preparation of the book.

contributors

editors

Susan Koch: RN, MN (Research), RCNT, Bachelor Educational Studies, Dip Professional Studies, FRCNA, FAAG. Senior Lecturer, Gerontic Nursing, School of Nursing, La Trobe University, Melbourne, Victoria. Susan commenced nursing at Glasgow Royal Infirmary, Scotland, in 1975. She completed her Bachelor of Educational Studies at the University of Stirling in 1988 and a Master of Nursing (Research) in 1995 at RMIT, Melbourne. At present she is undertaking her PhD at La Trobe University. Her clinical experience, research and teaching have been predominantly in aged care. Her funded research projects include restraint use, work with people with dementia and their carers, and reminiscence. Susan has presented her work at conferences and through publications, both nationally and internationally. She has also worked with Residential Care Rights and the Office of the Public Advocate resolving care issues involving the use of restraints on older people in residential care.

Sally Garratt: RN, Cert Midwifery, Dip App Sc (Nurse Ed), BEd, MScN (Colorado), FRCNA. Associate Professor, School of Nursing, La Trobe University, Melbourne, Victoria. Director of Nursing Education, Elanora, Vision Australia Foundation, Melbourne, Victoria. Sally began her nursing career at the Launceston General Hospital, Tasmania, and completed her midwifery at the Queen Victoria Memorial Hospital, Melbourne. She was awarded a W K Kellogg Foundation scholarship to study in North America and completed a Master of Science program at the University of Colorado. She has undertaken research in the area of human environment interaction, especially in dementia care. Sally has presented over 60 papers and undertaken numerous consultancies.

authors

Jennifer Abbey: PhD, FRCNA. Director, Advanced Health Care Management, Bribie Island, Queensland. Jennifer has been involved in aged care as a practitioner and educator for over two decades. Her research has been focused on the culture of residential aged care, particularly how that culture impinges on palliative care and the treatment of people with dementia. Her main interest is in combining theory and practice to assist in the realities of day-to-day care. She has been an invited speaker at national and international conferences on this subject. She sees advanced specialist practice as essential for gerontic nurses as they take greater responsibility for planning and implementing care for the aged.

Emeritus Professor Margaret Bennett: AM RN, Dip Nurse Ed, BA, BSc (Hons), PhD, FRCNA. Currently, President of the Nurses Board of Victoria and formerly Dean, Faculty of Nursing, RMIT, Melbourne. Margaret has many years of clinical nursing experience gained in both Australia and Canada. She has been involved in nursing education for over 30 years, initially in hospital-based programs for both division 1 and division 2 nurses and later at the post-graduate level in community nursing, and in diploma, degree and doctoral programs in the higher education sector. Margaret undertook both an under-graduate degree and her doctoral program at Monash University, with a research focus on clinical decision making in nursing. Following this period of study, she was active in facilitating the growth of nursing research in Australia, serving on numerous committees and teaching at various levels in the area. She has pub-lished widely in both Australia and overseas, especially in relation to clinical judgment. She has served on numerous committees in nursing and education and was a member of the ministerial taskforce on nurse practitioners in Victo-ria and chair of the Victorian Nurse Recruitment & Retention Committee in 2000.

Yvonne Coleman: B App Sc (Food Science & Nutrition), Grad Dip Diet, Grad Dip Health Education & Promotion. Yvonne is the founding principal of Nutrition Consultants Australia, and provides a consultancy service to nursing homes. One of her primary concerns is the consumption of polypharmacy in the elderly, and its effects on their nutritional status. Frustration at the lack of readily available information in this important area led Yvonne to publish the authori-tative *Drug-Nutrient Interactions: The Manual* (1998, Nutrition Consultants Australia, Melbourne). Yvonne was the chief dietitian at the Mount Eliza Centre, a position she held for more than eleven years. During this time she has developed a special interest in aged care. A current primary interest is the contribution of nutrition to falls. Previously Yvonne worked in the United Arab Emirates for a one year contract and, as a new graduate, she developed the dietetics service in East Gippsland. Yvonne believes that much of the debility associated with ageing has a strong nutritional component, and contributes to problems including frailty, falls, confusion, constipation, poor wound healing, and infections.

Elery Hamilton Smith: AM, Professor and Honorary Research Fellow at the Lincoln Gerontology Centre, La Trobe University, Melbourne. Elery has 50 years of experience in community work, social-environmental research and planning, teaching at Phillip Institute of Technology, Melbourne, and working across some 25 countries. In 1991, his long-standing interest in the leisure interests of older people led him to join with Sally Garratt in an extensive and continuing research program on the nature of dementia and the best ways of providing care for people with a dementing illness. Their research leads to a new understanding of dementia as a personal and social response to brain damage, which in turn opens up new and optimistic possibilities in the care of those affected.

Associate Professor Michael Hazelton: Associate Professor and Head of School of Nursing at Curtin University of Technology, Perth, WA. He gained a general nursing certificate in New South Wales in 1977 and a psychiatric nursing certificate, also in New South Wales, in 1981. Michael also holds Bachelor of Arts, Master of Arts and PhD qualifications in history, education and sociology from Macquarie University, Sydney. He moved to Perth in 1998 following nine years in Tasmania. Michael is also the current editor of the Australian and New Zealand Journal of Mental Health Nursing.

Susan Kurrle: MBBS, Dip Ger Med. Director and Senior Staff Specialist, Rehabilitation and Aged Care Service, Hornsby Ku-Ring-Gai, Hospital and Community Health Services, Hornsby, New South Wales. Susan is a medical practitioner with post-graduate qualifications in geriatric medicine. She has worked with the elderly for 20 years and has been involved in work and research in elder abuse for the past ten years. Apart from elder abuse, her major research interests are in the areas of dementia and hip fracture prevention. She is a board member of the NSW Alzheimer's Association, a director of the National Seniors Association and the Hammond Care Group, and has been a professional member of the NSW Guardianship Tribunal since 1992.

Dr Antonia (Anne) van Loon: RN, Dip Sc CHN, BN, MN (Research), PhD, MRCNA. Antonia grew up in Adelaide and completed her training to become a registered nurse at the Royal Adelaide Hospital in 1977. She continued her formal nursing studies at the Flinders University of South Australia, completing a Diploma in Applied Science in Community Health Nursing in 1984, a Bachelor of Nursing in 1987, and a Master of Nursing Research in 1995. Antonia submitted her doctoral dissertation in 1999, entitled 'Creating a conceptual model of faith community nursing in Australia'.

Richard Osborn: BSc, Dip Ed, Dip Aud, M Ed, M Aud SA (CC). Richard is an audiologist and educator. He is employed as the Director, Education and Consultancies, at Vision Australia Foundation. Over the past ten years, he has established and developed audiology and aural rehabilitation services for people with dual sensory loss at Vision Australia Foundation. He has also been involved in the development of rehabilitation services for people with general clinical impairment and blindness. He is a frequent presenter at conferences and seminars and has published over 20 articles in professional journals.

Wendy-Mae Rapson: B App Sci (Speech Pathology), M Sp Ed. Wendy-Mae is a speech pathologist and educator working in aged care and private practice. She is employed as an ageing and sensory loss specialist by Vision Australia Foundation and the Royal Freemasons' Homes of Victoria. She has presented papers at conferences in the area of ageing and sensory loss and is involved in the presentation of staff and care giver communication training programs.

Professor Marilyn Ray: RN, PhD, CTN, CNAA, BSN (Colorado), MS (Colorado), MA (Canada). Professor, Florida Atlantic University, College of Nursing, Boca Raton, Florida. Marilyn received her doctorate in Transcultural Nursing from the University of Utah. In 1990, she received a Fellowship to Australia where she lectured in transcultural caring and qualitative research methods at several colleges, universities and hospitals. Marilyn recently retired as a colonel after 30 years of service with the United States Air Force Reserve Nurse Corps. As a certified transcultural nurse, she has published widely in caring in organisational cultures, caring theory and inquiry development, transcultural caring, complexity science and transcultural ethics. She is on the editorial board of the Journal of Transcultural Nursing. Marilyn's research has revolved around technological, ethical and economic issues related to caring in complex organisations. Her current research, using both qualitative and quantitative research methods, relates to the study of the nurse–patient relationship as an economic resource, and how the economics of health and managed care are affecting the practice and administration of nursing. She is active in local, national and international educational activities.

Bridget Sutherland: Twenty-seven years experience as a furnishing consultant and a close involvement with aged care projects provides the background for Bridget's specialisation in the aged care environment. She and her husband are founding directors (1972) of Mondo Furniture Pty Ltd, a company which designs and manufactures contract furniture and has developed special expertise in designing for the comfort and safety of elderly people. Bridget has also promoted the ideal of 'adaptable housing'—a concept of housing designed to suit people at all stages of life. She was invited to submit to the 1997 Victorian Parliamentary 'Inquiry into Planning for Positive Ageing' and her recommendation that a model 'house for all ages' be constructed was received as a Victorian Government International Year of the Older Person project.

the foundation for assessment

what is assessment?

Margaret Bennett

chapter summary

This chapter will define some of the terms used in the assessment processes and detail the steps of problem solving through a critical and reflective examination of issues, situations and experiences. These skills are all necessary for effective clinical decision making. The chapter will highlight the importance of patterns in clinical decision making and suggest strategies to assist you in increasing the range of thinking patterns that you use. It will also draw to your attention the importance of intuition and how the expert nurse uses this thinking process when making effective decisions.

objectives

After reading and reflecting on this chapter, you will be:

- able to differentiate the terms *assessment, clinical judgment, clinical decision making* and *problem solving*
- able to build the types of assessment patterns that are essential in the making of clinical decisions
- aware of, and able to use effectively, the processes of intuition that characterise an expert clinician
- aware of the importance of immediate and accurate recording of your assessment
- able to, with practice, apply problem-solving skills in the assessment of older people who require nursing care.

introduction

To illustrate the expertise necessary for developing problem-solving skills in effective clinical decision making, consider the following scenario:

'You know Holmes, your assessment was "spot-on" for Mrs Bartlett. Your diagnosis enabled us to develop a set of behaviours for her that have reduced her anxiety and made her more content. She is now eating and sleeping normally and is no longer disruptive to other residents. How on earth did you do it?' Thus spoke Nurse Watson, a new graduate, to Nurse Holmes, a clinical nurse specialist in gerontological nursing.

'I could say it was elementary, my dear Watson, but it was not. Assessment is rather like detective work. It involves gathering information or looking for clues, making sense of the information, putting it into a pattern and labelling that pattern; that is, making a nursing diagnosis. We both gathered the same information, but the patterns into which we put it were different. I suspect that you missed the importance of some pieces of information and so you forced all the pieces into those patterns you know. I, on the other hand, from my experience, placed more importance on some of the information and therefore found that it fitted better into a different pattern from yours. I guess at this stage, I also know of many more patterns than you do, as I have been working in this area of nursing for many years. So you see, it's not only clinical knowledge that's important in assessment, but also experience.'

'Does that mean that time will make me as good an assessor as you?', asked Watson. 'Time alone is not important', replied Holmes. 'Rather, it's how you build up patterns from what you observe. You need to know what information to collect and then what to do with it. You also need to reflect on your own thinking and how you are processing the information that you observe. It's therefore a combination of clinical knowledge, decision-making skills and careful reflection on your experience. I'll help you by showing you how I arrive at my assessments, but you'll see that this is not always how the books tell you to do it, nor is it always as logical as my namesake would want it! In fact, I use intuition to great effect. I see I have shocked you, but perhaps after you have worked with me for a while you will understand better.'

Nurse Holmes has revealed to Nurse Watson how she became an expert in the assessment of older people. It involved four aspects:

1 Developing problem-solving skills that are integral to the clinical decisions or judgments that must be made.

2 Developing a clinical knowledge base. This involves drawing on what is learnt in various courses such as an undergraduate degree in nursing and masters degree in gerontological nursing. It necessitates reading widely, particularly books and journals; systematically surfing the Internet; and attending study days and conferences to keep up with the latest developments in gerontological nursing and related areas. It further requires that the nurse be part of a team undertaking evidence-based research into practice to ensure that the nursing care being given is the best available.

3 Reflecting on experience and by so doing making sense of the vast amount of information that must be processed in order to make a clinical judgment. Such information is put into patterns so that judgments can be made quickly, accurately and efficiently.

4 Using intuition as well as logical processes.

what is clinical decision making?

Before examining the process of assessment, it is important to look at it in the broader context of clinical judgment. Firstly, clinical practice requires the clinician to make judgments about those in care. Clinical decision making relates to the judgments we must make about the older people in our care. For the purposes of this chapter, the terms clinical judgment and clinical decision making will be used interchangeably. For an effective assessment, we must decide on the information we need to collect about the person, how it will be processed and what diagnosis we will make (see Figure 1.1).

Once having made an assessment, we must then decide on the nursing actions required, how we will provide these actions, whether the older person also requires care from other heath professionals, whether we should delegate some aspects of care, how we will determine to whom to delegate, how successful our nursing care has been and if not why not, and what we can do to make our care better. These are just a few of the decisions we have to make on a daily basis. Some of these decisions are simple, some are highly complex; some we make alone, others require us to consult the older person and/or their significant others, our nursing colleagues, or other health professionals. The calibre of our decisions is inextricably linked to the quality of the care we provide.

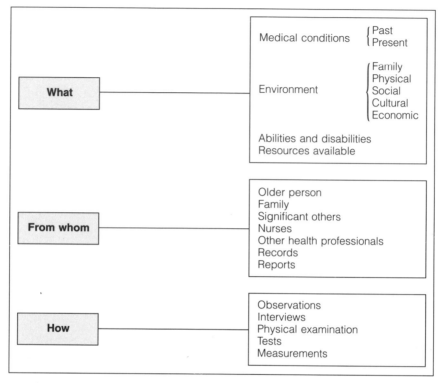

Figure 1.1: *Information collected for nursing history*

What then is decision making? Despite the amount of research that has occurred (or perhaps because of it) there is not agreement as to what it is, how it should be done or how to teach people to do it. It tends to be seen as a problem-solving exercise in which the decision maker must choose between two or more possible courses of action. For our purposes, decision making will be considered to be a complex, usually multifaceted problem solving operation. The word problem seems to offend some people, as not all that we encounter in nursing relates to problems. However, for our purposes it will mean an *unmet need*. Our task is to identify this need and then determine the *goals* that are necessary in order to have the need met. Older people present to us with needs that they cannot meet and for which some form of nursing intervention is necessary to help that person either meet the need themselves or have others meet it for them.

what is the problem-solving process?

There are many models of problem-solving processes. Some of these contain many steps, described in fine detail. At the other extreme only two steps are considered, namely, diagnosis and management. If you want to understand the various models of decision making as applied to the clinical field, a useful place to commence is any book that gives you an overview of such models. There are many on library shelves, but a useful one might be an Australian text by Thomas, Wearing and Bennett (1991). Tanner (1986, 1987 and 1993), an American nurse, has written some overviews of clinical decision making in nursing. Such overviews also provide useful references to pursue in the areas of your interest.

In this chapter, a model of problem solving using eight steps will be described (see Figure 1.2). These steps are those that are found in many decision-making models and reflect those in the so-called hypothetico-deductive model of scientific reasoning (eg, Hempel, 1968), Bruner, Goodnow and Austin's Concept Attainment Theory (1956) as well as the application of these models by Thomas (1989), and those contained in nursing texts such as Griffith and Christensen (1982) and Marriner (1983). These steps may actually occur together, but it is convenient to describe them as a sequence of events. The steps can apply to decision making in any context, but we will apply them in the clinical field of nursing of older people.

1 collect relevant information (take a nursing history)

In order to identify problems (ie, needs that are unmet), as much relevant data as possible must be collected. We need facts relating to the present and the past. The information collected will relate to all aspects of the older person: current and past medical conditions; family, social, cultural, environmental and economic situations; abilities and disabilities—physical, behavioural, environmental, social, cultural and economic—and the resources available to the older person. We collect this information from the older person, from family and significant others, from available records and reports, and from nurses and other health professionals. We also collect information from our own observation, interviews, physical examinations and various measurements. In this collection phase, it is important that we consider the facts as facts only and not rush into putting our own interpretation on them. It is very

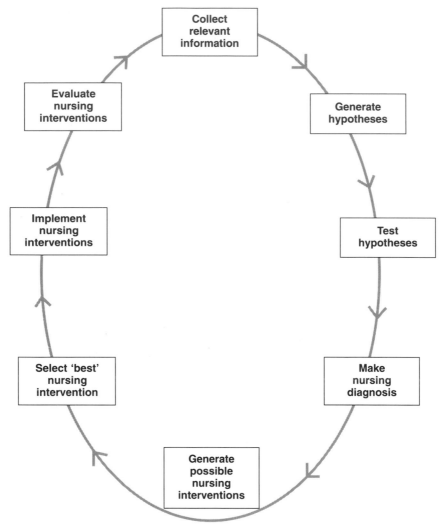

Figure 1.2: *Steps in problem-solving*

easy to do this, but we can later miss important information by not giving our full attention to the facts, as they become known to us.

When the facts are exhausted, or are not available, then opinions are sought from the older person, family, significant others, nurses and other health professionals where necessary. Such opinions can provide us with valuable information beyond the facts. Thus the information we collect is both objective and subjective, with the latter giving depth to the former. All the information, both objective and subjective, is recorded as the older person's history. It is important to ensure that the objective and subjective data are clearly recorded as such and the facts not confused with opinion.

2 generate hypotheses

As we are collecting this information, ideas start forming in our minds. We entertain 'best guesses' as to what the problem might be. These best guesses are called hypotheses and our task is to explore each hypothesis to see which is the most likely to apply to this particular older person. For example, a thin older woman might tell us that she has been eating only bread and jam for most of her meals. She lives alone and the first hypothesis might be that she needs some health teaching about diet. However, there might be other problems—economic, medical (relating to swallowing for example), or an underlying psychosocial problem relating to eating alone. Having formed some hypotheses, we then need to define and delimit the problem and so the next step is to test the hypotheses.

3 test hypotheses

The information that we now collect is concerned with confirming or refuting hypotheses. This step requires the sorting of relevant information into patterns associated with the hypotheses. We have established a number of patterns with the information we have already collected. We must now determine if the information we require to complete this pattern is available and if it fits well. If it does not, then we will need to rethink our patterns. In this process, some hypotheses are eliminated and those that remain form clear patterns (we will look more closely at pattern development later, as it is a crucial part of the process). During this step, the information we have collected is recognised, sorted and classified into patterns or categories. We are analysing the information and, in so doing, using clinical knowledge, analytical skills and drawing on experience. Once we have satisfied ourselves that we have sorted all the information into patterns or categories, it remains to label the problem or make nursing diagnoses.

4 label the problem (make nursing diagnoses)

The labels may vary, but in the assessment phase of a clinical judgment, we have a diagnosis. If you look up this word in a dictionary you will find that it is derived from two Greek words: *dia* meaning thorough or precise and *gnosis* meaning to know or recognise. It is an interesting word for, as we know, diagnosis in nursing and medicine is sometimes far from precise. However, we use the word to mean a process of recognising, sorting and classifying phenomena into discrete categories (or patterns) to which labels are attached (Thomas, Wearing and Bennett, 1991). The process of diagnosis is the same for all health care professionals, but the content matter and the labels differ. Nurses, doctors and physiotherapists, for example, all diagnose different aspects of health and illness, for which they are accountable. The language for each set of diagnoses is different and unique to the profession. One such system used in nursing is that provided by the North American Nursing Diagnosis Association (NANDA), a system that has universal application and is being used in Australia in some areas of the aged care sector. This is unique and, while it requires us to work hard in understanding the labels, nonetheless the processes underlying the labels are sound. We need a labelling system so that we can communicate effectively within our profession.

Once the diagnosis is determined it is important to clarify your diagnosis with the older person and/or their family. Once clarification confirms the data, the assessment phase is complete. In completing this process, we have collected, analysed and labelled relevant information about the older person. We have completed the diagnosis phase of problem solving. We must then pass into the management phase. Having sorted out the information to make an assessment of the person in care, it is necessary to work out how to solve the problem. The first step is to generate possible solutions to identified problems, or interventions for diagnosis.

5 generate possible solutions to identified problems (nursing interventions)

For any problem, there is usually more than one solution. Initially as many solutions as possible will be considered. Some of these solutions, in our case nursing interventions, will arise out of the clinical knowledge base. We need to ensure that we are up to date with the latest in nursing care so that we are able to provide the full range of possible solutions that are available. Each of these possible solutions needs to be considered in terms of its consequences and acceptability to the clients. Apply the 'if then test' (eg, if I use this strategy for Mrs Bartlett, then these consequences are likely to occur). Once tested, the nursing interventions can be arranged in a rank order, so that you can then select the best solution.

6 select the 'best solution' (optimum nursing intervention)

This step requires not only a sound clinical knowledge, but an understanding of the older person as well. What might be best for one person might not work with another person. We also need to remember that a solution that appears 'best' in theory might not be possible in the setting in which we are working—we do all have some constraints upon us and must work within these. However, the guiding principle must be what is best for this particular older person and then to pursue this goal. Having decided on the 'best' solution it remains to implement the course of action.

7 implement a course of action (nursing intervention)

This may require you to take the action yourself, or to delegate it to others, depending on which is the more appropriate for this person. If you delegate it to another, then you are still accountable for the outcome of the action. You must be sure that the person to whom you delegate has both the knowledge and skills to carry it out effectively and efficiently. You must monitor closely its outcomes. It is also important that the plan of the nursing interventions is recorded in the care plan and that progress towards the established goal is recorded and monitored. Where progress is not satisfactory, the assessment process will need to be repeated on an ongoing basis. Having monitored it closely, you will then need to evaluate the effectiveness of the action(s).

8 evaluate the effectiveness of action(s) or interventions

Has the un-met need been met? Is it being met in the most effective and efficient way? Have you recorded it in such a way that the outcomes are clearly identified in the care plan? Was your assessment accurate? Was it the correct diagnosis? How closely does the action that you have taken reflect the assessment? If it was successful, why was it successful? If not, why not? Where the desired outcomes have not been achieved, then the process of assessment will need to be repeated. You will also need to reflect on the whole process. This process of reflection is an essential part of evaluation. It is through this that we build up the range of patterns that characterise the expert nurse—an issue that will be considered later.

As indicated above, the steps may occur together and they tend to go in a circle. As we monitor and evaluate, we may find that we need more information, we need to revise our hypotheses, change our diagnoses, seek more information and change our courses of action. It is a living, dynamic, cyclic process. It is therefore essential that, at each step of the way, we record what has been decided. This will ensure those who care for this older person can provide continuity of care. It will also enable us to know how much time must be provided for nursing care for this older person and hence the resources required. It will also provide a clear record of the effectiveness of our care and show what a difference nursing can make to the older people in our care.

From the above, it can be seen that assessment requires us to collect relevant information, analyse that information (ie, recognise it, sort it and classify it into patterns that are the 'best fit' for the information) and then to label that pattern or category. A diagnosis is therefore the end point of assessment. The management phase requires us to plan the nursing care that is to be provided, by determining what is the best goal to set to ensure that the un-met need is met for the older person. Following this, it is important to devise the nursing strategies or interventions that will help the older person to reach that goal in the most effective and efficient manner. These strategies must then be put into action (ie, the plan implemented), and then the progress of the older person is monitored and the plan evaluated.

problem solving and the nursing process

You may have recognised the terms assessment, planning, implementation and evaluation as being those described in what Yura and Walsh (1988) originally called the nursing process. They later added diagnosis as a separate step between assessment and planning. This nursing process was introduced as an attempt to apply problem solving in an orderly and systematic way to nursing. It was popular for many years. It also received considerable criticism, but the fact remains that it did make us think about the way we use problem-solving processes in our nursing care.

From the above, you can recognise the steps that you use in assessment and management of your clients. The focus in this book is on assessment and, as indicated above, assessment consists of the collection of information, its analysis and, following analysis, the labelling of the categories or patterns that have been derived. In nursing terms this means that we take a nursing history, analyse the information and reach our diagnoses. Nurses are generally very good at collecting information, but not always as skilled in its analysis. The key to good analysis lies in how we build and use patterns.

pattern building and recognition

what is a pattern?

The amount of information we receive each day is enormous and we need to develop ways of dealing with it to enable us to cope, without information overload. As suggested above, we tend to form patterns of information to help us make sense of the world. What are patterns? They can be described as an organisation of elements to form a coherent entity. Think of the many patterns that you carry with you. When you think of an older person, what elements are organised to make your pattern? As a nurse, your pattern might be confined to what you see daily in the hostel or nursing home where you work. An older person to you may be someone who is frail, unable to meet all the demands of daily living, and struggling to adapt to a life away from his or her own home and family. To me, an older person is someone who is healthy, living to capacity within any limitations, and enjoying the luxury of retirement— although at a pace a little slower than previously. To a nurse working in the community, a different pattern might emerge: one centring on how a person manages in his or her own home environment coping with chronic illness. Thus, three different people dealing with aged people may have different patterns, depending largely on the context in which they find themselves.

Here is an exercise for you. What is your pattern for dementia? Is it different from that held by members of your own family? Ask them. You should expect their patterns to differ form yours, as your experience is likely to be more extensive. But is your pattern the same as that of your colleagues? Ask them. Did you find that their patterns varied? How could this be? You all work in the same context; however, the secret to pattern building lies in our level of knowledge and experience. Our socialisation and formation of values also shape our learning. When you were a student nurse, no doubt you learnt the various lists of symptoms for medical diagnoses, or the defining characteristics for nursing diagnoses. However, those for whom you were caring more often than not had the effrontery to appear without some of these clues and others did not fit the textbook pattern. What you did was to build up your own patterns that matched what you were seeing in the workplace. There is some research available that shows how new nurses, or novices as Benner calls them, have different patterns from the expert nurse (you can read about this in Benner's book *From Novice to Expert*, 1984, as well as in other research studies that support Benner's findings). It is interesting to examine these different patterns.

novice versus expert patterns

In essence, novices see the elements as separate entities, usually as they are presented in the textbooks. Thus, the pattern for novices would be A + B + C + D + E + F and the whole pattern would be the sum of these parts. If any of these elements were missing, then the diagnosis could not be made. More experienced nurses group the entities into configurations and recognise relationships between the elements. Thus, to make a diagnosis, more experienced nurses might just want to see A, C and E in a particular relationship. The whole is therefore more than the sum of the parts—the relationships between the parts are also considered. Sometimes there may be a part G that is not in the textbook, but from experience it is known to usually be present in a particular relationship with the other elements. If, as an experienced nurse, you reflect on your own decision making, you will find that this is so.

Novices also rely on rules and principles that are evident in the textbooks, whereas experienced nurses may use rules of thumb that they have built up from experience. These rules of thumb are known as heuristics and we will return to these presently. Experienced nurses will also tend to look at the whole pattern and will be alerted to small and subtle changes in this pattern. Sometimes these changes are so small they do not reach a conscious level. Thus, experienced nurses may not only rely on logic and rationality as do novices, but may also use intuition—an issue we will discuss later. Experienced nurses will be faster, process less irrelevant information and be more accurate in diagnosis than novices. How do we get to this level of pattern formation?

To answer this question we need to remember that nursing is both a science and an art. Among the characteristics of science are those of objectivity, precision, logic and rationality. In rational decision making, all the information available is processed in a logical manner. For this we rely heavily on clinical knowledge that can be measured and that has been researched as to its accuracy and validity. These are the facts that we need to collect as part of the data collection process and these facts tend to fit into patterns easily. For example, where *Mycobacterium tuberculosis* has been isolated, we have no hesitation in diagnosing tuberculosis, as we know that this micro-organism causes tuberculosis. On the other hand, in the art of nursing, we use our own personal knowledge, based on experience; and we might use biases, hunches and intuition in our pattern recognition.

intuition

Benner suggests that expert nurses are differentiated from other levels of nurse by their use of intuition. What is intuition? Dictionaries define it thus:

> . . . immediate apprehension of the mind without reasoning. (Oxford Dictionary)

> . . . direct perception of truth, facts etc. independently of any reasoning process. (Macquarie Dictionary)

Benner (1984) defines it as 'initially by-passing critical analysis' and 'understanding without reasoning'.

All these definitions suggest that whatever intuition is, it occurs at a level below conscious awareness. Within our own experience we all have examples of intuition. We have had 'gut feelings' about our clients. It may be a feeling of uneasiness, or not feeling 'right'. We just know we have to act. If anyone asks us why we acted in this way, we reply to the effect that we do not know why, but we knew it was right. On reflection, we can sometimes work out why we acted as we did, but not always. However, the important thing is that we need to recognise intuition as a characteristic that does separate the more experienced, reflective nurse from the novice. It was what Nurse Holmes was using effectively in the scenario at the beginning of this chapter. In their insightful article on intuition, Benner and Tanner (1987) give us some ideas of how we build up our patterns at a level below consciousness. They highlight a number of heuristics (rules of thumb) that have been identified in the clinical decision-making research. We will largely use the work of Benner and Tanner here, but apply it to the aged care setting wherever possible.

heuristics

representativeness

This occurs when we use only a small number of all the possible clues available to us to make a decision. What happens is that, over time, we see the outcome of our decision-making process associated with a certain outcome, based on this limited amount of information. For example, a nurse might 'know' that in order for Parkinson's disease to be diagnosed, all that needs to be present is a particular gait which the nurse might have difficulty describing, and a particular facial feature. Now, this may not seem enough for you, but this experienced nurse has built up this pattern over many years, and more often than not it is accurate. The nurse might not be able to articulate that this is what she or he is working on, but nonetheless this pattern exists.

configurality

This one we have already mentioned. It occurs when patterns are developed that concentrate on the relationship between the clues, rather than on each element individually. Benner and Tanner (1987) provide an excellent example. They were interested in the fact that nurses were able to interpret outcomes from Swan-Ganz waveforms more accurately than physicians. What they discovered was that, where the physicians tended to concentrate on each element of the waveform separately, the nurses, from their experience, tended to build up a picture of the waveforms as a whole. When subtle changes occurred in this overall waveform they came to associate it with a particular outcome. Thus, the elements *per se* were not the focus of attention, but rather, the relationships between them in an overall pattern. If you think about your practice, you may note that you too may look at relationships between things rather than the elements themselves. You may also respond to subtle changes in an overall pattern, sometimes so subtle as to be below the level of conscious awareness.

common-sense understandings

Sometimes expert nurses match more than they know to an existing pattern. This might sound a little fanciful. How can we do this? Look back at the definition of intuition. More is going on than we are consciously aware of. You will develop a pattern of the older person as a whole, taking into account their language, culture, physiology, usual patterns of behaviour, coping mechanisms and emotions. However, the expert will also consider the taken-for-granted matters such as how the older person looks, talks, feels, even eats breakfast. Every nurse has access to this common-sense information, but it is the expert who sees its relevance in recognising subtle trends in that person's health picture. For example, an older person putting salt on her egg with her left hand one morning, when her usual pattern is the right hand, may not seem of any importance. However, it is a subtle change in the normal pattern and an expert nurse will follow this up, perhaps without even being conscious of why. Think about some of your own examples here. You may bring aspects of your care to consciousness that you were not aware of before.

case matching

One of the features of assessment is the matching of a present pattern to ones of the past. More often than not, this is done below the level of conscious awareness. For example, Mrs Bartlett has a strange reaction to Ventolin. It is different from the usual, but the nurse might recall another client, Mr Christides, who had a similar reaction many years ago. Just thinking of Mr Christides enables the nurse to gain access to this pattern. The two reactions are matched and a new pattern is now confirmed. It will be used wherever this particular unusual reaction occurs. This approach helps the nurse to select the most relevant clients for comparison with a new pattern. The wider the nurse's experience, the more such patterns can be used. In some situations it might be only one aspect of the whole pattern that does not fit the usual case, or it might be a missing link for a new pattern.

salience

Given the amount of information that we are called upon to process, the expert learns to recognise some aspects of a pattern that stand out as features from a background of information. Experience helps us to use this strategy and enables us to place more importance on some elements, or some relationships, without having to process all the information. We look for the features that we consider stand out. Sometimes, however, this can take quite an amount of searching out. It takes not only a deep knowledge of the client as a person, his or her culture, and social and environmental aspects, but the intuitive perception to allow the salient feature to emerge. It might become clear from a chance remark of the older person or family member. Once it is found, it always stands out and we can use it as an established pattern.

metaphor and imagery

The decisions that we make below the level of conscious awareness may be difficult to describe. Sometimes the only recourse that we have is to use a metaphor or an analogy—something that creates an image of what it is we are trying to describe. Listen to the language that your experienced colleagues use when attempting to describe something that they know is right, but do not really know why. Such language might be disturbing to the scientist, but it reflects not a lack of knowledge or judgment, but rather the inexactitude of the situation and the complexity that is required to make sense out of ambiguous information.

Thus, there are a number of rules of thumb or heuristics that we use in our clinical judgments. See if you can think of examples from your own experience that match those above. You may well be surprised at how often your thought processes are not the logical, ordered ones that you think they should be.

conclusion

Assessment is an exercise in problem solving. It enables us to identify problems by collecting relevant information, analysing it into categories or patterns and then attaching a label to that pattern. The range of patterns that you have access to reflects your level of expertise in assessment. Patterns are built up from knowledge and experience. Knowledge and technology are constantly changing and all nurses need continuing education to keep their knowledge and practice current. However, experience also helps to build the patterns that you use. More patterns can be built when you reflect on your practice and identify those patterns. Remember, though, that not all the patterns that you use are at a level of conscious awareness. It is your use of intuition that also helps to make you an expert in the area. Thus, for effective assessment, you need to know how to make clinical decisions using the steps of problem solving processes. You also need to ensure that your knowledge is up to date and comprehensive. Further, you need to reflect on your practice and thus build a wide range of patterns. However, you need to acknowledge that some of your patterns have been built up through intuition. All these aspects are important in the process of assessment.

Finally, you need to record accurately the steps of your assessment in your nursing notes. This ensures not only continuity of care but has an effect on the amount of funding that your facility receives. You might also like to consider that just as you are a role model for clinical practice, you should also role model your thinking processes—especially when you are using patterns that have been built up from your experience, as well as your knowledge. This is what Nurse Holmes, a self-confessed user of intuition, was going to do with Nurse Watson, who was still a novice with restricted knowledge and experience and a limited range of patterns.

study questions

1 What information is recorded on the older person's nursing history?
2 How is information analysed in order to arrive at a nursing diagnosis?
3 You have been asked above to think about some of the patterns you have and how these differ from those of other professionals and your family. You are now also asked to reflect on your own practice and how you have built up some of the common patterns you use. How many heuristics (rules of thumb) did you use to build these patterns?
4 Can you think of some examples of your own use of intuition? What was the outcome of such use? (You might find that the outcomes of intuition are not always as you expected, but that is part of your own experience and needs to be reflected upon.)
5 How would you go about role modelling your assessment thought processes to a student of nursing?

references

Benner, P. (1984), *From Novice to Expert*, Addison-Wesley Publishing Co., California.

Benner, P. and Tanner, C. A. (1987), 'How expert nurses use intuition', *American Journal of Nursing*, January, pp. 23–31.

Bruner, J. S., Goodnow, J. J. and Austin, G. A. (1956), *A Study of Thinking*, John Wiley & Sons, New York.

Griffith, J. W. and Christensen, P. J. (1982), *Nursing Process: Application of Theories, Frameworks and Models*, Mosby Co., St Louis, Missouri.

Hempel, J. A. (1968), *Philosophy of Mind*, Prentice-Hall, Englewood Cliffs, New Jersey.

Marriner, A. (1983), *The Nursing Process: A Scientific Approach to Care*, 3rd edn, Mosby Co., St Louis, Missouri.

Tanner, C. A. (1986), 'Research on clinical judgment' in W. L. Holzemer (ed.), *Review of Research in Nursing Education*, Vol. 1, National League for Nursing, San Francisco.

Tanner, C. A. (1987), 'Theoretical perspectives on research on clinical judgment' in K. J. Hannah, M. Reimer, W. C. Mills and S. Letourneau (eds), *Clinical Judgment and Decision-making: The Future with Nursing Diagnosis*, John Wiley & Sons, New York.

Tanner, C. A. (1993), 'Rethinking clinical judgment' in N. L. Diekelmann and M. L. Rather, *Transforming RN Education: Dialogue and Debate*, National League of Nursing, San Francisco.

Thomas, S. A. (1989), 'Clinical decision making' in N. King and A. G. Remenyi (eds), *Psychology for the Health Sciences*, Nelson Wadsworth, Melbourne.

Thomas, S., Wearing, A. and Bennett, M. (1991), *Clinical Decision-making for Nurses and Health Professionals*, Harcourt Brace Jovanovich, Sydney.

Yura, H. B. and Walsh, M. B. (1988), *The Nursing Process*, 5th edn, Appleton-Century-Crofts, New York.

holistic assessment

Susan Koch

chapter summary

This chapter informs the reader of the necessity for holistic assessment, including assessment of the family. The chapter is written to assist you in helping older people, where possible, to take control of their own health and personal care. This can be undertaken when we have a shared understanding of the older people and recognise that, like us, they are complex individuals. Using a simple approach, you are introduced to documenting how the individual and the family can be holistically assessed using a genogram and ecomap.

objectives

After reading and reflecting on this chapter you will be:

- able to identify the importance of integrating the individual and the family in undertaking a holistic assessment
- aware of the effective use of genograms and ecomaps as assessment tools
- able to undertake a family assessment using a genogram and an ecomap.

introduction

According to Sappington and Kelley (1996), 'to provide holistic care, nurses must attempt to view the world through the eyes of the person'. In Chapter 1, it was noted that assessment provides the basis for planning and implementing care. However, the quality of this care is contingent on the nurse's ability to adequately assess. Before undertaking an assessment of an older person, the nurse must have a thorough understanding of the physical, psychological, social, environmental and pathological effects of ageing. This knowledge provides a good grounding on which to make available information to the older person, and/or to their family, in order that the best care decisions can be made. In recent years, older people requiring our assistance have seen an increase in the use of technology to assist in medical diagnoses and treatment. They are also better informed, which may lead to conflict between the older person and health care workers. Therefore, there is a requirement for nurses to be able to answer the questions asked of them and to be prepared to be questioned by the older person and/or their family.

In holistic assessment, the nurse should initially explore the older person's strengths, as this takes the focus away from disease. Since many older people cannot be 'cured' from growing old and frail, it is important to identify their strengths and strategies they have used previously to assist them in coping with changes. It is also important to identify how the person perceives the concerns that require them to seek assistance with their health and well-being. We also need to identify what care they desire and what they do not want.

Maslow's (1968) hierarchy of needs has been used as a basis for care; however, the hierarchy of needs may not truly reflect what the person desires. The hierarchy of needs commences with the basic physical needs, safety needs, social needs, esteem needs, cognitive needs to, finally, self-actualisation. When assessing these needs, we can see that in relation to physical needs, the changes associated with ageing and the predisposition to increased dependency will affect this, the most basic of needs. Safety needs can be affected by the ageing process, reduction of mobility and reduced sensory abilities. The losses associated with normal ageing can have an effect on meeting the social needs of the older person; this may be related to loss of a spouse, change of accommodation, or loss of belongings. Changes in self-esteem can result from a change in family or community roles (here we may include our society's negative stereotyping of older people as affecting an older generation's perception of themselves and their contribution to society). In relation to cognitive needs, many myths about ageing may have an effect on whether or not the needs of older people are met. Opportunities for learning or creativity may be restricted as it may be considered inappropriate to provide such stimulus, or that older people are not capable of such activities. Finally, the need for self actualisation may not be seen as an imperative, especially when the physical needs may be overwhelming for the health care workers. Yet it is a normal aspect of human development to be challenged, and to continually learn and develop as an individual. Development does not just stop at a certain age or when a specific medical diagnosis has been given.

While Maslow's hierarchy may be useful, there is a tendency for health care workers to implement this model in an accumulative manner. That is, when the basic needs are met, the higher needs will be dealt with. However, this may not be how the older person perceives their needs. The need for cognitive stimulation may be the key factor in successful implementation of care. It is important to commence the assessment by asking the person what their goals are and what they want to achieve with your assistance. For the older person who can no longer articulate their goals or needs, the health professional then draws on data collected from others. This may include family members, friends, other health professionals, clergy or other people involved in the life of the older person. When commencing the assessment process, it may be useful to consider what quality of life means to the individual. For some, the components of quality of life include living without fear, having meaning in your life, and contributing to society or your family (Blenkner, 1957).

On examining what quality of life is for the individual, it may be difficult to see how these can be attained through the normal delivery of health care, yet if we are to restore and maintain quality of life these components and others should be included in all aspects of holistic assessment. An integral part of holistic care is allowing the person to make their own decisions and to decide what risks they want to take regarding their care.

models of care

We can begin to see that assessing all facets of an individual requires skill, expertise and time if the task is to be done well. Undertaking an assessment using a model of care will assist in providing a framework on which to document the findings of an assessment.

Several nursing models of care have been developed to assist nurses in the assessment process. Neuman's (1989) systems model of nursing contends that we cannot fully understand people and their behaviour unless we also understand the relationship between them and their environment. Orem's (1971) self-care model uses the personal contribution to health and wellbeing rather than their state of ill-health. Roper's (1979) 'activities of living' model identifies key qualities true of all human beings, focusing on the observable behaviours accompanying them.

Whichever model is used, nurses are required to emphasise the importance of holistic assessment and care delivered to an individual and their significant others through a shared understanding of the person requiring care.

holistic assessment of the older person

Assessment of the older person commences with finding out:

- Who they are: name, age, marital status, place of birth, employment, family role, what it was like growing up.
- What have been the biggest changes they have seen.
- Who their family is; where they grew up; how many are in their family; whether they have an extended family; whether 'pet' names were used, who used them, and whether they are still alive.
- Who their friends and confidantes are.
- What work they undertook: paid or unpaid; what their role was at work; what it was like; whether they enjoyed it; where they worked (eg, overseas or interstate); whether they had more than one job; what their pay was.
- What they would like to do now they are getting older.
- What makes them happy.
- What brings them contentment.
- What frightens them and what would reduce that fear.
- What makes them feel good about themselves. What they would say were their achievements in life and how could these be used to assist them now.
- What contribution would they like to continue making to society.

Documenting the responses to these questions lends itself to the use of genograms and ecomaps. These tools are more commonly used in family assessment; however, as the older person is part of a family it would seem logical that this approach can be used.

the older person and the family

Changing demographic and social trends make it imperative to respond to the complex and growing health care needs of our ageing citizens and their families. Older adults as individuals vary in their past life experiences as well as in their current physical, financial and living circumstances. Likewise, families vary greatly in their ethnicity, histories, structures, coping styles, values, resources, living circumstances and needs.

In aged care, whether residential or community-based, nurses need to work in partnership with the family to maintain optimal functioning, restore health and prevent and/or reduce the effects of illness in the older members. To accomplish this, nurses should assist families and provide care to their older loved ones that promotes the optimal health and functioning of *all* members, regardless of their age. Nurses are required to use adept, reflective communication while assisting family members to define and clarify any issues that may have arisen within their family roles.

Sometimes, when the demands of family caring exceed the family's resources and compromise their wellbeing, nurses may need to assist the family in choosing the most appropriate care. To ensure the optimum outcome, nurses should focus on assessment, planning, management, intervention and evaluation of care, not only for the individual concerned but also for the family as a unit.

As stated earlier, nurses will find it helpful if they have an in-depth understanding of the biological sciences, the ageing process and the physical aspects of health and illness, as this will allow them to monitor physical wellbeing and assist family members to participate and understand care procedures.

Age is commonly accompanied by one or more chronic health problems. An older person may experience a loss of independence by limitations in the ability to function and carry out self-care activities. Many individuals over the age of 65 experience a period of dependence and a need for care before reaching the end of life. More women than men are in need of help because older women are more likely to be widowed and to live alone. They have less income than elderly men and they have more chronic health problems such as arthritis, osteoporosis and diabetes (AARP, 1991; Biegal, Shore and Gordon, 1984; Courtney and Price, 1999).

The family, not the formal health care system, provides 80 to 90 per cent of care to their elderly members, including medical and nursing care, personal services such as transportation and help with household tasks and shopping (Brody, 1985) (Courtney and Price, 1999). The family responds to emergencies, provides acute care and assistance, and initiates and maintains links with the formal care system as necessary. Also, the more frail an older member becomes, the more responsibility for care the family assumes (Biegal and Blum, 1990). Despite this evidence, there is a lingering myth among many nurses that family members—especially adult children—do not provide care for elderly family members when they need it but instead rely on formal services such as nursing homes. In truth, adult children are providing more assistance and more comprehensive care to their elderly parents than in the 'good old days' (Brody, 1985; O'Neill and Sorenson, 1991).

family development

Families are like individuals in that each has a life cycle with predictable developmental stages and changes. The changes that families experience over time are like those in a kaleidoscope. Events, whether the accumulation of small changes or a major stressor, result in the creation of a new pattern from the existing components of family life. Some changes are subtle while others are more dramatic, but the changing patterns unfold progressively and uni-directionally.

Until the occurrence of a stressor event or crisis that demands change, families usually maintain fairly stable patterns of interaction over time. Events that demand change take two forms, normative and non-normative. Normative changes or transitions are those expected, somewhat predictable, maturational life events such as marriage, birth of the first child, retirement and death of a spouse in old age. Although these are expected changes, a period of floundering or crisis may occur until adjustment is achieved. Non-normative crises, on the other hand, are not predicted or expected and may occur with little warning. Examples include the diagnosis of a serious, chronic illness or the accidental death of a family member.

assessment of the family

Transitions within older families occur when roles and responsibilities start to shift across the generations. Middle-aged children often find their ageing parents coming to them for emotional support, advice and other forms of help. This may occur at a time when their own children are leaving home, the family's financial resources are stretched to pay for university tuition and the mother is returning full-time to the work force. For the older generation, the changes brought by retirement, possible loss of income and physical decline may bring fear and trepidation. Reaching out to their children for help is often a disturbing and even humiliating experience. As much as they need the help, they may have great difficulty in asking for it.

As elderly members begin to develop signs of physical or cognitive decline that threaten their independence and capacity for self-care, several things are likely to happen. There may be a shift in the traditional hierarchical structure as parental authority and influence decline, which brings shifts in roles, responsibilities and boundaries. Adult children are confronted with the filial crisis, a concept introduced by Blenkner (1957) in an attempt to explain the experience of adult children when care of their parents becomes necessary. The children are forced to face the fact that their belief that their parents will be there forever is a fantasy. Instead of continuing to be the recipients of parental nurturance, they must become the nurturing ones, both to their parents and to the younger generation. Middle-aged children's sense of loss and distress may be intensified because they must admit to their own mortality as their ageing parents must acknowledge their decline, need for help and loss of independence (King, Bonacci and Wynne, 1990).

genograms and ecomaps as nursing assessment tools

Drawing family trees is an ancient practice, on which family physicians have elaborated for clinical use, as a means to obtain and display genetic and medical information about a family. Genograms have also been used by psychologists to examine patterns of interactions within families. Nurses, too, are beginning to use the genogram, but with an emphasis on the social, behavioural and cultural aspects of a family. (Wright and Leahey, 1994).

Similarly, the ecomap has its strengths in its visual impact. As with the genogram, family members can actively participate in the development of an ecomap during an interview or family assessment. Ecomaps clearly display the family members' contact with others, including internal and external family members, friends, social contacts and services (Wright and Leahey, 1994). Genograms and ecomaps can convey a large amount of information in a visual format. When one considers the number of words needed to express the facts genograms and ecomaps can represent, it becomes clear how simple and useful these tools are (ibid.).

genograms

To create a genogram, one begins by drawing the basic family structure and those identified as significant others as far back as the older person can remember. This is often only as far back as the grandparents, and older people need to be reassured that they are not expected to remember distant relatives and specific dates. Begin the interview by discussing easy, factual matters. Once the basic skeleton has been drawn, you can continue adding significant information. Information is gathered in three categories: demographic, functional status and resources and critical events or dynamic changes. Figure 2.1 shows standard genogram symbols and Figure 2.2 shows a basic genogram format.

demographic information

Demographic information involves a factual database that includes age, present location, major role, occupation and retirement status, major health problems, educational level, and, for deceased individuals on the genogram, the date and cause of death. Careful recording of all dates

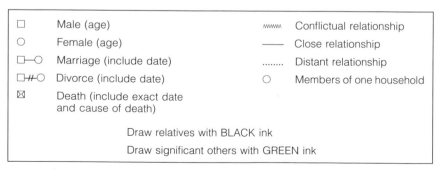

Figure 2.1: *Standard genogram symbols*

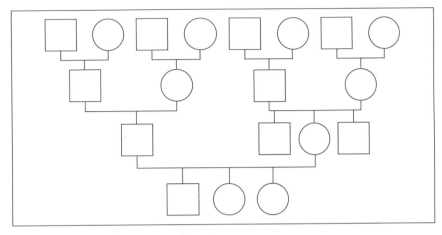

Figure 2.2: *Basic genogram format*

will identify pertinent data that may indicate areas of note. For example, knowing the exact day and month of the death of a significant other may enable plans to be made to cope with anniversary reactions (Hansen and Boyd, 1996).

functional and resource information

Obtaining functional and resource information involves questioning the older person about their present functional health status in the context of available and significant intra-personal and environmental resources. Resources are considered to enhance or distract from a level of health; therefore, this information is vital.

critical events

Critical events and/or dynamic changes are those events the client perceives as significant. It is helpful to begin exploring this area with a general question and then to proceed to more specific questions concerning successes, losses, and transitions in physical, emotional, social and financial aspects of life. Critical events may be recorded either in the margin of the genogram or, if necessary, on an attached sheet of paper.

Genograms can become very complex, but it is important to keep them as simple and clear as possible; too much data will cause confusion and the purpose of the genogram will be lost. The major advantage of the genogram is its graphic format. The nurse can glance at it and get an immediate picture of the situation without going through a large amount of notes, and critical information can be flagged and quickly seen.

The information gathered through the genogram can play a critical role in the development and implementation of preventive health plans and health promotion activities. The goal is to describe the client accurately and to organise the data in such a way that strategies with which to protect, promote and maintain the health of the client are apparent.

The completed genogram should not become the property of the nurse. Clients should be encouraged to share it with family members and friends so that the therapeutic process can continue.

ecomaps

Family genograms are an integral part of ecomaps. The genogram is placed in the centre circle of the ecomap, which is labelled 'Family' (see Figure 2.3). The outer circles represent people and agencies that are significant to the family. Lines are drawn between the older person, family members and the outer circles. Straight lines indicate strong connections, dotted lines indicate tenuous connections and slashed lines indicate stressful relations. The wider the line, the stronger the tie.

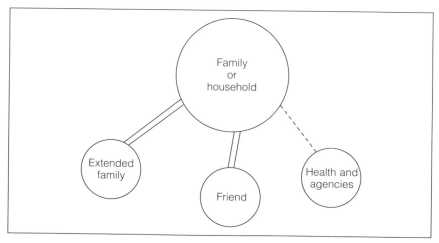

Figure 2.3: *Format of an ecomap (adapted from Wright and Leahey, 2000)*

uses and benefits of genograms and ecomaps

The uses and benefits of genograms and ecomaps in assessing and inter-vening with elderly clients are many. They provide a ready framework for establishing non-threatening communication. Older people are often afraid of health care professionals and, for some, their exposure to the health care system has been limited to, or thought of, as a last resort. Thus, a way to establish a supportive, caring relationship is extremely important.

Genograms and ecomaps create a powerful experience for everyone involved, including the nurse. They provide a highly organised and visually effective method of gathering and displaying information, and communicating this information to the client and to other health care professionals. They can serve as tools to stimulate reminiscing and to further growth and self-esteem in the older person.

conclusion

This chapter has highlighted the necessity for holistic assessment that must include the family. We must encourage older people, where possi-ble, to take control of their own health and personal care. This can be undertaken when we have a shared understanding of people and recog-nise that, like us, they are complex individuals. The genogram and ecomap can provide a powerful experience for everyone involved, including the nurse. Not only do they provide valuable information, they can also serve as tools to stimulate reminiscing. We must use every available resource that will assist in the personal development of the individual and promoting positive self-esteem for those for whom we care.

activities

Use the case study below for the following activities:

1   Using the case study, complete a genogram and an ecomap for Sara.
2   Suggest strategies you could use to improve relationships between staff and Sara's family.

case study: Sara

Seventy-eight-year-old Sara received a diagnosis of dementia over five years ago. The exact type is unknown but her symptoms correspond with those found in Alzheimer's disease. She has been separated from her husband for many years (exact details unknown). Because of her deteriorating condition, Sara moved in with her daughter's family. As Sara was unable to provide any information, her family provided the details to be inserted into a genogram and ecomap; these are as follows.

Sara married Theo in 1949, when she was 29. She and Theo migrated from Greece soon after their marriage, which meant leaving all of their family behind and arriving in Melbourne knowing no-one.

She was a solitary person and had no real close friends. Sara worked as an office cleaner. Her working hours were 9 pm until 11 pm and 7 am until 9 am. She did this type of work most of her working life and retired at the age of 65.

Sara enjoyed gardening, walking and cleaning. Sadly, she was constantly abused physically, mentally, emotionally, sexually and financially by Theo. Sara often slept with one or more of the children while they were at home. The children considered this was her way of trying to protect them from the father, though he never abused them. Sara has four children: Angelina (50), Alan (48), Sara (45) and Greg (40). All are married and all except Sara have children.

Theo left Sara some 35 years ago and has never contributed, either financially or emotionally, to the support of the children. The family have no contact with their father or their mother's family in Greece.

Angelina has two children and lives with her husband Eric. Angelina took Sara to live with her when Sara's condition started deteriorating. After several years of caring for her mother, Angelina's siblings became concerned for Angelina's health and insisted she go on holiday for a rest and agreed to share the care for their mother. While Angelina was away, the family considered Sara's care needs were too much for Angelina to deal with and arranged for Sara to be placed in extended care.

Angelina returned from holiday to find that her mother had been placed in care and is having great difficulty in coming to terms with the decisions made in her absence. She phones the facility for reports on her mother's health at various times of the day, visits every day for around three hours and constantly challenges staff regarding the care of her mother. The staff of the facility consider this behaviour unnecessary and disruptive to the routine of the facility.

Angelina maintains contact with her siblings and appears to enjoy a close relationship with all of them. Decisions are made in a collaborative way and each member of the family has input, including the grandchildren.

From the ecomap we can determine that family relationships are strong. However, the relationship between the aged care facility and the family is fairly negative. The next stage of the assessment process would be to determine why this negative relationship exists and develop strategies as to how this can be overcome.

references

American Association of Retired Persons (AARP) (1991), *Profile of Older Americans*, American Association of Retired Persons and the Administration of Aging, US Department of Health and Human Services, Washington D.C.

Biegal, D. E. and Blum, A. (1990), *Ageing and Caregiving: Theory, Research, and Policy*, Sage Publications, Newbury Park, CA.

Biegal, D. E., Shore, B. and Gordon, E. (1984), *Building Support Networks for the Elderly: Theory and Applications*, Sage Publications, Newbury Park, CA.

Blenkner, M. (1957), Positive Factors in the Initial Interview in Family Case-work. *Dissertation Abstract*, 17, pp. 2061–2.

Brody, E. M. (1985), 'Parent care as a normative family stress', *Gerontologist* 25, pp. 19–29.

Courtney, M. and Price, G. (1999), in R. Nay and S. Garratt (eds), 'Funding and policy in residential care' *Nursing Older People: Issues and Innovations*, MacLennan & Petty, Sydney, pp. 18–39.

Duvall, D. E. and Miller, B. C. (1985), *Marriage and Family Development*, 6th edn, Harper & Row, New York.

Hansen, S. and Boyd, S. (1996), *Family Health Care Nursing: Theory, Practice and Research*, F. A. Davis, Philadelphia, pp. 330–48.

Kendig, H. and Brooke, L. (1999), 'Social perspectives on community nursing practice' in R. Nay and S. Garratt (eds), *Nursing Older People: Issues and Innovations*, MacLennan & Petty, Sydney, pp. 135–50.

King, D. A., Bonacci, D. D. and Wynne, L. C. (1990), 'Families of cognitively impaired elders: Helping adult children confront the final crises', *Clinical Gerontologist*, 103–15.

Maslow, A. (1968), *Toward a Psychology of Being*, Van Nostrand Reinhold, Princeton, NJ.

Neuman, M. A. (1989), 'The spirit of nursing', *Holistic Nursing Practice* 3, (3), pp. 1–6.

O'Neill, C. and Sorenson, E. S. (1991), 'Home care of the elderly. A family perspective', *Advances in Nursing Science Journal* (4), pp. 38–7.

Orem, D. (1971), *Nursing: Concepts of Practice*, McGraw Hill, New York.

Roper, N. (1979), 'Nursing based on a model of living', in M. M. Colledge and D. Jones, *Readings in Nursing*, Churchill Livingstone, London.

Sappington, J. and Kelley, J. H. (1996), 'Modeling and role-modeling theory: A case study of holistic care', *Journal of Holistic Nursing*, Jun 14(2), pp. 130–41.

Wright, L. M. and Leahey, M. (1994), *Nurses and Families: A Guide to Family Assessment and Intervention*, 2nd edn, F. A. Davis, Philadelphia.

Wright, L. M. and Leahey, M. (2000), *Nurses and Families: A Guide to Family Assessment and Intervention*, 3rd edn, F. A. Davis, Philadelphia.

chapter 3

transcultural assessment

Marilyn Ray

chapter summary

This chapter explores the world of older adults from a cultural viewpoint by examining the concept of culture, the cultural context of ageing, cultural ideas of health and illness, transcultural nursing, and the application of Ray's Transcultural Gerontologic Assessment Tool (see Appendix 3.1). The meaning of transcultural gerontological nursing will be elucidated through a case study that reveals the culture and late-life developmental and health issues of an older Vietnamese man.

objectives

After reading and reflecting on this chapter, you will be:

- aware of the significance of transcultural nursing
- able to analyse the meaning of culturally competent care
- aware of the patterns of meaning associated with cultural development
- able to apply the Ray transcultural gerontological assessment tool in assessing older people.

introduction

Assessing ageing from culturally diverse perspectives provides the foundation for effective nursing care in contemporary nursing practice. Transcultural assessment of older adults in any health care environment, from home, clinics, hospitals to nursing homes, offers challenges for learning and enhancing the lives of both clients and caregivers. Older people from culturally and linguistically diverse backgrounds face unique developmental tasks as well as expected and unexpected life events which must be evaluated from the way these individuals view their own health situations (Cavanaugh, 1993; Cutillo-Schmitter, 1993, 1996; Grossman, 1994). Immigrants from diverse groups, as well as Indigenous people, often recapture the distinctive patterns and meanings associated with their own cultures as they age. This reminiscence plays a vital role in how they respond to interventions and outcomes of care.

Transcultural assessment is the search for culturally relevant information and the understanding of how the reality of illness, health and wellbeing is filtered through the older person's cultural lens. The health care professional must understand the importance of the cultural lens in providing culturally competent care. Transcultural assessment integrates sociocultural content by including the health beliefs, preferences and practices of diverse groups of individuals with biopsychological and developmental evaluation.

The health of Australia's Aboriginal and Torres Strait Islander population is poor and life expectancy is less than that of the white population.. While governments have endeavoured to address the reasons for this over the years, there is still a lack of understanding by health professionals of the impact of cultural differences within the Indigenous groups. The fact that the cultural heritage of Indigenous people is different from tribe to tribe across the country is often not recognised. In Victoria and parts of New South Wales, the Aboriginal culture is Koorie (Anderson, 1988). In other areas of Australia, the Indigenous people will have different cultural backgrounds and languages. To assume all Indigenous cultural groups are the same is as erroneous as assuming all Italian or all Greek groups are the same. There may be a common understanding of lifestyle and some understanding of language but the cultural beliefs and values that create the meaning of existence will vary. The term *transcultural* illuminates the importance of a shared intercultural relationship between the professional and the client.

the concept of culture

The concept of culture is the foundation for understanding the cultural meanings attached to the concepts health and illness, transcultural nursing, and transcultural assessment of older adults. Many anthropological theories of culture exist, ranging from holism, structural-functionalism, adaptation, behaviourism, cognition to symbolic interactionism and shared meaning systems (Geertz, 1973; Keesing, 1981). Definitions of culture vary. Over time, theories of culture have changed from an emphasis on objective, material culture to a more subjective approach grounded in meaning. Today, culture is generally thought of as a system of learned and shared knowledge, beliefs, customs, and symbols or patterns of meaning that is communicated, developed, and transmitted to other members of a group (Geertz, 1973). Symbols and icons are objects that have developed cultural meaning and assist people to function and integrate a world view or belief system. Social structural characteristics reflect the objective structure of culture. Objective functional forms that create the social structure (eg, kinship, religious, political, technological, legal and economic systems) play a significant role in helping us to understand patterns of meaning.

Human organisation revolves around biological variation, ethnicity, gender, sexual orientation, and growth and development. Culture and ethnicity have been distinguished, although the terms are often used interchangeably. Ethnicity is a group's identity, based on common factors such as religion, nationality, place of birth or shared cultural patterns, and refers to social differentiation based on cultural criteria—culture, social status and social support. Most importantly, ethnicity refers to a shared identity (Ebersole and Hess, 1998). Race initially referred to biological origin and physical appearance but now social meaning related to patterns of living is affixed to the definition. As globalisation and multiculturalism become more widespread through cultural expansion, intercultural communication, and interracial marriage and progeny, more research will be conducted to better capture the nature of human variability and lineage among diverse people of the world (Overbey, 1997).

Multiculturalism is dynamic and complex, contextual and public, as is the meaning of life itself (DeSantis, 1997; Fuller, 1996). When many people interact, either between members of the same cultural group or with others outside a group, complex meanings emerge. As the political support for multiculturalism increases, especially in the west, so too will the need to sustain cultural identities, particularly as people age.

the cultural context of ageing

Each year, the net balance of the world's older people increases dramatically in both developing and developed countries. Women constitute more than half of the aged population in virtually all parts of the world on which data are available (Sokolovsky, 1990, p. 17). A global perspective on the status and support of the aged is on the horizon. A truly cross-cultural comparative gerontology seeks to uncover key variables to gain an understanding of ageing. There is a distinction between cross-national and cross-cultural perspectives. Cross-national views take as their unit of analysis the nation-state, and encompass whole countries by measuring demographic, interactional and health related variables. Cross-cultural views of older people, on the other hand, focus on smaller scale societies or communities within nation-states. These small scale societies can be compared by focusing on the differences and similarities among cultures that contribute to theory advancement, and alternative strategies can be suggested for developing a better environment in which to grow old (Sokolovsky, 1990).

The cultural context in which people grow old creates a varied reality of what ageing means. The cultural systems of nation-states or individual cultures (values, perceptions, human relationships, and the social organisation or socially constructed behaviours) all contribute to the way ageing is defined. Culture only exists in relation to the contextual framework in which human beings find themselves. Western cultures have more varied understandings in relation to the aged than non-industrialised cultures. The normative family in most western countries has changed owing to declining birth rates, smaller families, and the lengthening of life expectancy resulting in more generations living at the same time—the verticalisation of the family or the concept of the multi-generational family structure (Agren, 1992; Hargrave and Anderson, 1992). 'Intimacy at a distance' (living apart but maintaining a close relationship) has become a strong value of western families. In the United States and other western cultures, the values of self-determination, independence, individualism and privacy are accentuated. These values, while inherently admirable in some circles within western cultures, have contributed to social isolation of the elderly and may be considered threatening to family life because they undermine intergenerational relationships (Simic, 1987). However, the strength of the belief in independence prevails even in old age. For example, what the American aged fear most is 'demeaning dependence' on their children or other kin (Simic, 1987, p. 94). Maintaining control of lifestyle decisions and exercising choice to sustain independence for older adults in western countries is of critical importance (Agren, 1992). The western paradox of the need for closeness and the need for privacy provides opportunities to explore with individuals how best to form supportive environments for older people.

In non-western cultures, research demonstrates that the cumulative effect of the important roles the elderly play in kinship and communal relationships, such as the transmission of knowledge, spiritual leadership, and the direction of communal beliefs, is a cultural context in which the elderly are well supported (Sokolovsky, 1990).

Of special concern among the cross-cultural comparative views of being old is encountering the darker side of ageing—various types of non-supportive and even death-hastening behaviours against the elderly. Cultural distinctions have been drawn between the later stages of the human life—the oldest old and the frail elderly—and the earlier phases within the ageing cycle—the intact and fully functioning elderly. When older people are classified as 'frail' or 'feeble' (ie, unable to carry out the most basic tasks), geronticide or death-hastening is most frequently discussed or applied (Glascock, 1983).

Sokolovsky and Sokolovsky (1983) report that the potential security and quality of life of older people is maximised when cultures facilitate and value both their community and kin roles, and these arenas of interaction are mutually supportive rather than constructed as separate entities. Where does that leave people who have emigrated from non-western cultures to western cultures? Studies show that international migrants are no more likely to experience psychological instability than other groups. There is also no evidence to support claims of poorer mental health in ethnic minorities, but it has been found that they suffer from racially discriminatory practices in treatment. Studies show that race, ethnicity and class represent stronger forms of influence on the experience of old age than being old itself (Bytheway et al., 1989). The following section focuses on two main aspects of the transcultural assessment of ageing: cultural health and illness and transcultural nursing.

cultural beliefs and practices in health and illness

Beliefs and practices about illness and health are central attributes of all human cultures (Helman, 1994; Brown, 1998). Health is intrinsically connected to the way in which people in a culture construct reality and give and find meaning in their lives, to the way in which communities are created and administered (Cohen, 1989), and to the way in which professional health care expertise functions in a society. Health and illness, therefore, are not simply consequences of an individual's physical nature (Nader and Maretzki, 1973). People construct their reality in terms of mental patterns characteristic of their image of the body, mind, spirit, family, community and culture. The social organisation of health and illness in the society (primarily the formal or dominant health care system) determines the way in which people are recognised as sick or well and the ways in which illness is dealt with by health care professionals (Helman, 1994).

medicine and nursing

Medicine and nursing can be considered as cultures within their own right; however, medicine has been viewed more as a biomedical science than a culture (Embree, 1994; Lupton, 1994; Ray, 1989) and nursing has been viewed more in terms of its role as a handmaiden to physicians. Recently, the idea of the nurse as an advocate for the patient has been supported in western cultures. Both medicine and nursing are infused with values, beliefs and attitudes about illness and health which have come primarily from the dominant cultures within which they exist. In western cultures, generally speaking, health is not intimately connected to the authenticity of the relationship between health care professional and client, to the way in which the forces of nature behave or to the way in which communities function, for example, as in eastern cultures where health is related to harmony. For the most part, the health professions (especially medicine) govern and influence the way in which people will confront illness and receive care.

transcultural nursing

Leininger (1991a, 1995, 1997) launched the discipline of transcultural nursing and designed a theory of cultural care diversity and universality to generate knowledge and apply the knowledge in practice to provide culturally relevant care to clients and their families. 'Transcultural nursing is a specialised discipline focused on care meanings, values, and practices within specific cultural contexts to discover and explain ways that *culturally constituted care* contributes to the health and wellbeing of people, or helps people face death and disabilities' (Leininger, 1997, p. 342). The purpose of Leininger's theory of cultural care is to identify human care differences or commonalities and comprehend the impact of the social structure (political, economic, legal, technological, educational and religious) and cultural worldviews on individuals and families and on nursing care decisions and actions. In addition, the transcultural field developed so that health care personnel could become more aware of their own beliefs, values and treatment practices and how their values inadvertently or intentionally are imposed on people of other cultures (Leininger 1991b; Purnell and Paulanka, 1998).

An important element of Leininger's theory is the interrelationship between the generic or 'folk' culture of the individual and the professional system of the nurse. The folk or generic culture is a specific assembly of manifestations and physical signs that have a range of symbolic meanings—moral, social or psychological—for those who suffer from them. For example, folk illnesses are learned and can be hot and cold diseases, the evil eye, heart distress, social stresses and depression, sorcery, witchcraft and so on, that are expressed in physical or psychological forms. Television, the internet, literature, and the social structure or dominant ideologies of a culture also influence the way illness is perceived (Helman, 1994). Knowledge of how folk illnesses are generated is important for nurses so that collaborative and negotiative health care decisions between health care professionals and clients can be effectively made. Professional nurses see themselves as the primary guardians of their patients through advocacy or cultural brokerage (Jezewski, 1993). Cultural brokerage is now necessary as a form of nursing to facilitate access to ever changing health care systems. The culture broker or advocate has to negotiate, on behalf of the client, with the physician, other health professionals, insurance companies, and state or national governments to represent the client's needs and mediate for culturally relevant health care and subsequently better health, especially for ageing minorities.

transcultural assessment of the aged

An effective way to provide nursing care for older adults is not only to attempt to understand people's customs, the caregivers who are designated to provide care (such as particular family members), and the rituals that sustain health or wellbeing, but also the way in which these activities appertain to the social system. Ray's Transcultural Geronto-logic Assessment Tool (see Appendix 3.1), based in part on social structural characteristics identified in the works of Leininger (1991a) and Ray (1994), is a technique to assess and understand the care needs of older adults (see also Figure 3.1). What is important in this approach to transcultural nursing assessment is the recognition that the nurse also is a cultural being and brings his or her values, attitudes and behaviour to the nurse–patient relationship. Successful evaluation of ageing people from whatever culture depends upon the caring relationship and an appreciation of the power of culture—symbols, rituals, and patterns of health care—in the healing process. Contemporary nursing therefore requires a discerning awareness of the significance of health and illness from clients' worldviews. The following case study of an older Vietnamese man (adapted in part from a portrait of the Vietnamese by Farrales, 1996 and Shanahan and Brayshaw, 1995) is used to illustrate a transcultural nursing situation to assist with assessment and preparation for the delivery of culturally competent care. The information presented for critical thinking and decision making is not necessarily a one-time-only assessment but is to be considered over time as the nurse

1   Discovery and understanding of the 'cultural self' for nurses and clients and its meaning in health and illness.
2   Knowledge of activities of daily living (ADL) and personal time construction and how they are managed.
3   Older adults may resort to their traditional beliefs and practices when encountering new developmental, physical, emotional and spiritual challenges.
4   Stories of older adults reveal the significance of their lives and cultures.
5   Families of older adults may engage their own familial cultural healing powers.
6   Intergenerational conflict about ways of life, religion and health may emerge.
7   Caregivers and family members of older adults may resort to abuse of older adults if misunderstanding occurs related to issues of cultural illness and healing.
8   People from non-western cultures may give different cultural meanings to the ageing process.
9   The use of the terms *compliance* and *non-compliance* in the provision of culturally competent care needs to be examined by professional nurses.
10 Transcultural assessment means providing culturally relevant care for older adults.

Figure 3.1: *Overall issues or problems to be considered in the nursing care of older adults from different cultures*

continues in a caring relationship with the client. The case study is intended to be an interactive project wherein the professional nurse is invited to become fully involved by responding to the questions and applying Ray's Transcultural Gerontologic Assessment Tool.

case study: Mr Nguyen

Fiona, a public health nurse at a clinic in Adelaide, the capital of South Australia, is feeling the exhaustion of the day. She has returned from a home visit to a 75-year-old Vietnamese émigré of nearly 20 years to Australia named Mr Nguyen. Fiona has not had a great deal of experience caring for Vietnamese clients; however, she is now called upon to visit the client and develop a plan of care from her assessments. Mr Nguyen, recently widowed, lives with his daughter, Than, who was home briefly for the nursing visit. Than interpreted for Mr Nguyen because he is not fluent in English. Than is 30 years old and single and has lived in Adelaide since she was a child, when she arrived with her parents from Vietnam. She speaks English fluently. She is employed full time as a laboratory assistant in a pharmaceutical firm. (Fiona thought Than was very 'westernised' by the style of her clothes and the beliefs she shared about her life and her father's state of health and illness.) Two paternal uncles and their wives and their children live in Adelaide. Mr Nguyen's two sons and their families returned to live in Ho Chi Minh City, Vietnam, four years ago to start a business. Although part of a large Vietnamese population in Adelaide, Mr Nguyen has not participated with the group either for social functions or in day care settings. Mr Nguyen and his two brothers and their families exchange visits in Adelaide.

Mr Nguyen does not feel well and his health care problems have been worsening. He is suffering from congestive heart failure and arthritis, and is very thin, possibly due to inadequate nutrition over many years and perhaps since the beginning of the Vietnamese conflict in the 1960s. Mr Nguyen does not eat well although Than tries to prepare traditional meals with vegetables and rice which are his favourites. Often Mr Nguyen and Than eat quite late because Than has to work late three nights a week. Mr Nguyen has been experiencing greater congestion and has an irregular heart rate. He also experiences pain in his knees, hip and fingers. Mr Nguyen was given a prescription for Digoxin by the family doctor after he started having symptoms. Than said Mr Nguyen doesn't like to take the medication and misses a dose now and then. Than has explained to Mr Nguyen how important it is to take the medication. (Mr Nguyen seems to be in pain and appears to be sad.) When Fiona spoke with Than, she explained that all her father wants is to go home to Ho Chi Minh City. Mr Nguyen said he was lonely and he told his daughter that he wants to go home to die. Than said although he has been in Australia for 20 years, he longs for his homeland and reminisces about his life as a young boy. Mr Nguyen wants to be home and be with his sons and where he can practise his Buddhist beliefs and have the monks visit him as they did with his parents and grandparents. Empathising with Mr Nguyen's situation, Fiona is now grappling with a plan of care that will respect his culture and that of his family.

specific vietnamese cultural themes to consider

1 Identify the history of Vietnamese immigration, especially the immigration patterns of refugees.
2 Determine what language is spoken: Vietnamese dialects, French, Chinese.
3 Recognise a highly family oriented culture—use a family member as a consultant and interpreter if possible.
4 Recognise that the eldest son or father is usually the family spokesperson.
5 Limit touch (non-verbal communication) with older adults (this generation tends to be very modest).
6 Avoid direct eye contact with older adults.
7 Respect personal health information (be sensitive and softly spoken).
8 Explain the medication schedule with a family member of the older adult.
9 Learn about food preferences: most people prefer warm and soft food and rice with each meal; many Vietnamese may be lactose intolerant.
10 Recognise that older Vietnamese adults may be stoic with pain and may not report any problems unless asked by the nurse.
11 Acknowledge the stigma relating to mental illness (depression or sadness). Older Vietnamese adults may not seek help from professionals.
12 Acknowledge that older Vietnamese adults may not respond to problems until they are severe.
13 Appreciate that the person may believe in both biomedicine and traditional medicine (herbal, acupuncture and spiritual practices).
14 Recognise that older adults as patients often assume passive roles, and that the women in the family are usually responsible for caring roles.

15 Appreciate that older adults may prefer to die at home with dignity, with visits from monks. Cremation is preferred by Buddhists.

Answering the questions and applying the tool to the older adult and his family described in this case study demonstrates that gerontologic transcultural nursing assessment and planning is a mutual and collaborative enterprise. Integrating cultural concepts relating to the individual, family and the community facilitates an understanding of the meaning and significance of the cultural context of ageing.

conclusion

As more and more western populations are becoming multicultural and are ageing, the need for cultural competence in providing compassionate and holistic health care to the most vulnerable among us is necessary. Family, community, religion and history are important reference points for sustaining identity and self-worth for ageing adults of different cultural backgrounds to our own (Ebersole and Hess, 1998). Global changes based on rapid communication, devaluation of ageing people, destruction of traditional languages, economic competition and intergenerational discontinuities are threatening the process and meaning of growing old in world societies. Nurses have the interest, concern and knowledge to demonstrate leadership in the arena of transcultural aged care. Opportunities to meet the challenges at individual, local, national and international levels must be seized.

references

Agren, M. (1992), *Life at 85: A Study of Life Experiences and Adjustment of the Oldest Old*, University of Goteborg, Goteborg, Sweden.

Anderson, I. (1988), *Koorie Health in Koorie Hands*, Koorie Health Unit, Health Department, Melbourne.

Bytheway, B., Keil, T., Allatt, P. and Bryman, A. (1989), *Becoming and Being Old*, Sage Publications, London.

Brown, P. (ed.) (1998), *Understanding and Applying Medical Anthropology*, Mayfield Publishing Company, Mountain View, CA.

Cavanaugh, J. C. (1993), *Adult Development and Ageing*, Brooks/Cole Publishing Company, Pacific Grove, CA.

Cohen, A. (1989), *The Symbolic Construction of Community*, Routledge, London (original work published 1985).

Cutillo-Schmitter, T. (1993), 'Family assessment', in C. S. Fawcett, *Family Psychiatric Nursing*, Mosby Year Book, St Louis, Missouri.

Cutillo-Schmitter, T. (1996), 'Ageing: Broadening our view for improved nursing care', *Journal of Gerontological Nursing*, 7, pp. 31–42.

DeSantis, L. (1997), 'Building healthy communities with immigrants and refugees', *Journal of Transcultural Nursing*, 9(1), pp. 20–31.

Ebersole, P. and Hess, P. (1998), *Toward Healthy Ageing*, 5th edn, Mosby, St Louis, Missouri.

Embree, L. (1994), 'Reflection on the cultural disciplines', in M. Daniel and L. Embree (eds), *Phenomenology of the Cultural Disciplines*, Kluwer Academic Publishers, The Netherlands.

Farrales, S. (1996), 'Vietnamese', in J. Lipson, S. Dibble and P. Minarik (eds), *Culture and Nursing Care*, UCSF Nursing Press, San Francisco.

Fuller, J. (1996), 'Multicultural health care: Reconciling universalism and particularism', *Nursing Inquiry*, 4, pp. 153–9.

Geertz, C. (1973), *The Interpretation of Cultures: Selected Essays*, Basic Books, New York.

Glascock, A. (1983), 'Death-hastening behavior: An expansion of Eastwell's thesis', *American Anthropologist*, 85, pp. 417–21.

Grossman, D. (1994), 'Enhancing your "cultural competence"', *American Journal of Nursing*, 7, pp. 58–61.

Hargrave, T. D. and Anderson, W. T. (1992), *Finishing Well: Ageing and Reparation in the Intergenerational Family*, Brunner/Mazel Inc, New York.

Helman, C. (1994), *Culture, Health and Illness: An Introduction for Health Professionals*, 3rd edn, Butterworth-Heinemann, Oxford.

Jezewski, M. (1993), 'Culture brokering as a model for advocacy', *Nursing and Health Care*, 14(2), pp. 78–85.

Keesing, R. (1981), *Cultural Anthropology*, Holt, Rinehart & Winston, New York.

Leininger, M. (ed.) (1991a), *Culture Care Diversity and Universality: A Theory of Nursing*, National League for Nursing Press, New York.

Leininger, M. (1991b), 'Becoming aware of types of health practitioners and cultural imposition', *Journal of Transcultural Nursing*, 2(2), pp. 32–9. (Reprinted from Leininger, M. (1978), *Transcultural Nursing: Concepts, Theories and Practices*, J. Wiley & Sons, New York.)

Leininger, M. (1995), *Transcultural Nursing: Concepts, Theories, Research and Practice*, McGraw-Hill, Columbus, Ohio.

Leininger, M. (1997), 'Transcultural nursing research to transform nursing education and practice: 40 years', *Image: The Journal of Nursing Scholarship*, 29(4), pp. 341–54.

Lupton, D. (1994), *Medicine as Culture*, Sage Publications, London.

Nader, L. and Maretzki, T. (1973), *Cultural Illness and Health*, American Anthropological Association, Washington, DC.

Overbey, M. (1997), 'AAA tells feds to eliminate "race"', *Anthropology Newsletter*, 38(7), pp. 1 and 4.

Purnell, L. and Paulanka, B. (eds) (1998), *Transcultural Health Care*, F. A. Davis, Company, Philadelphia.

Ray, M. (1989), 'The theory of bureaucratic caring for nursing practice in the organizational culture', *Nursing Administration Quarterly*, 13(2), pp. 31–42.

Ray, M. (1994), 'Transcultural nursing ethics: A framework and model for transcultural ethical analysis', *Journal of Holistic Nursing*, 12(3), pp. 251–64.

Shanahan, M. and Brayshaw, D. L. (1995), 'Are nurses aware of the differing health care needs of Vietnamese patients?', *Journal of Advanced Nursing*, 22(3), pp. 456–64.

Simic, A. (1987), 'Ageing in the United States and Yugoslavia: Contrasting models on intergenerational relationships', in J. Sokolovsky (ed.), *Growing Old in Different Societies*, Copley, Acton, Massachusetts.

Sokolovsky, J. and Sokolovsky, J. (eds) (1983), 'Ageing and the aged in the third world, Part II', *Studies in Third World Societies*, No. 23, College of William and Mary, Williamsburg, Virginia.

Sokolovsky, J. (ed) (1990), *The Cultural Context of Ageing*, Bergin & Garvey Publishers, New York.

Appendix 3.1: Ray's transcultural gerontologic assessment tool

structural characteristics for assessment and culturally relevant care

questions for critical thinking to be used with Ray's tool

1 What are the cultural migration patterns of Vietnamese people in Australia?
2 Determine the biopsychological and spiritual components that place constraints on activities of daily living, personal time, and later life activities.
3 Determine the physical, nutritional, and pharmacological patterns for older adults with specific health problems.
4 What are the patterns of death and dying in Vietnamese culture?
5 What are the social or kinship factors of the Vietnamese? How do Vietnamese older adults relate to their children?
6 What are the communication patterns or styles of communication?
7 What are the indigenous cultural and health patterns and reminiscence patterns of Vietnamese that need to be taken into consideration by nurses?
8 What are the religious or spiritual patterns that need to be addressed?
9 What are the later life dependency needs of Vietnamese older adults and how would the professional enhance quality of life for this particular older adult?
10 How would the professional formulate a culturally relevant plan of care for this older adult and family?

assessment

Linguistic
- Determine the language or interpreter needs and the level of fluency in English.
- Discover the meaning of non-verbal gestures or behaviour.
- Identify with sensitivity when and how much information should be requested.

Social
- Act compassionately with the ageing person, family or significant others.
- Interact in a mutually collaborative manner to develop a trusting relationship.
- Identify the social needs of the ageing person, family or significant others.

Kinship
- Identify the family system of the client.
- Determine the current living situation (alone or with family members).
- Determine the extended family system.
- Identify the client's social and community support system.
- Discover the type of intergenerational relationships—harmonious or conflictual.
- Identify who makes health care and living arrangement decisions in the family.

Health care
- Identify the client's activities of daily living.
- Identify the client's personal time construction.
- Determine the client's perceptions of health problems, causes, and prognosis.

- Ascertain if there are physical or mental challenges to wellbeing.
- Ascertain if healers or practitioners within the culture are important and are used.
- Ask what, or if, medications (traditional or general) are used.
- Ask the client or family what makes him or her feel better.

Nutrition
- Request information regarding beliefs about foods and preferences.
- Identify if traditional foods are eaten.
- Determine if the hot-cold cultural system of food intake is used.

Spiritual
- Ask about religious and/or spiritual practices and their influence in health and healing.
- If appropriate, determine the client's and family's needs in relation to dying and death and the rituals practised in their particular religion or faith.

Economic
- Determine sensitively the socioeconomic status of the client.
- Determine the short- and long-term care economic, social support and living arrangement needs with the client and family.
- If, or when appropriate, arrange for economic support for the client and family.

Technological
- Ask about transportation—within and outside the home.
- Ask about the driving practices of the client, if any.
- Identify what technological equipment is in the home for communication, social support, and assistance with daily living.

Political
- Determine if there is or should be government intervention or assistance in the client's care.

Legal
- Determine what the legal needs of the client are in relation to culturally sensitive health care.
- Ask if the client has a will, living will, and/or power of attorney, if appropriate.

Educational
- Provide assistance with health care needs, based upon mutual evaluation of health and caring needs and patterns.
- Identify expectations for ongoing care, home care, nursing home care, hospitalisation, family and community support.
- Co-create a culturally relevant plan of care with the client and family.
- Mutually identify and develop a process for open, mutual communication and guidance for the provision of culturally relevant care.

chapter 4

assessing spiritual needs

Antonia (Anne) van Loon

chapter summary

This chapter introduces the concepts of spirituality, spiritual wellbeing, spiritual needs and spiritual care. The key spiritual needs that most nurses are likely to encounter when caring for older people include the need for meaning and purpose in life, love and belonging, hope, forgiveness, a relationship with God and transcendence of the human spirit. The chapter demonstrates the process of assessment of spiritual needs within the nursing process and provides two critical pathways to assist the decision-making process.

objectives

After reading and reflecting on this chapter, you will be able to:

- challenge your personal values and beliefs pertinent to spiritual assessment and whole-person care
- examine what constitutes spiritual needs in the older person and how these might be manifest by the older person
- explore a critical pathway for spiritual assessment
- identify the four methods of assessment used when assessing spiritual needs.

introduction

Models of nursing endorsing the whole person necessarily require assessment of needs within the physical, psychosocial and spiritual dimension of the person. This chapter discusses what a spiritual need is and why you should assess your client's spiritual needs. We look at two critical pathways that can be used to assess spiritual needs and demonstrate the nursing process of spiritual care. The chapter also challenges you to examine your personal perspective on the value of the person. When you become aware of your own value system, you are more able to assess the spiritual needs of others. The quality of your care improves dramatically when you assess and try to meet another person's spiritual needs, which in turn provides you with internal satisfaction and motivation. You are often providing spiritual care when you attend to the more 'ordinary' needs of people. For hidden in the ordinary is the nurse–client interface, which is the critical context of caring for the human spirit. Spiritual care is as much about how we interact and use ourselves as it is about specific nursing actions. This hidden aspect of nursing care is thus a taken-for-granted part of the ordinary activities of everyday nursing.

what do I mean by spirituality, spiritual wellbeing, spiritual needs and spiritual care?

There are many definitions of spirituality so let's begin by stating what I mean by spirituality. For the purpose of this chapter I will describe the person's spirit as the inner essence which is the basis of an individual's vital life principle. The spirit integrates the other dimensions of the body into a whole and transcends the body after death (Conrad, 1985; Carson, 1989). The spirit is the inner distinctive nature or qualities which makes the person the being they are (van Loon, 1995). Nurse participants in a research study conducted by van Loon (1995) said the spiritual dimension 'motivates and activates the mind and body' while the psychosocial dimension deals with 'mind and behaviour regulation of the developing person'. The spirit 'makes the person alive in a qualitative sense rather than a mechanical sense' (ibid., p. 111).

Religion and spirituality are not synonymous (Emblen, 1992).

However, many people structure their spiritual dimension within a religious framework which guides their moral and ethical value systems, and provides the rituals, practices, beliefs and history to nurture and develop their spiritual dimension (Dugan, 1987/88; Burkhardt, 1993).

The spirit enables the person to perceive a state of wellbeing from which they derive experiences of love, joy, hope, trust, forgiveness, inner peace, meaning and purpose in life (Barker, 1989; Burns, 1989). A spiritual need may be indicated by a lack of any of these intra-personal experiences, as these two nurses illustrate: '. . . lack of anything which is necessary to maintain the person's integrating life principles' (van Loon, 1995, p. 114). 'Factors which alienate or estrange the person from the centre of their own being, rendering them incapable of experiencing spiritual wellbeing' (ibid.). The spirit also enables a person to be in relationship with God (as defined by that person); thus a spiritual need is lack of any factor that enables this relationship to thrive (Fish and Shelly, 1988; van Loon, 1995). Research by Piles (1990) and Zerwekh (1993) found spiritual needs are manifest in psychosocial behaviours and emotions such as anger, despair, hopelessness, grief, anxiety, suffering, fear, pain, guilt and loss.

Spiritual care is always given in the context of the nurse–client relationship, which means you bring to the encounter your self. Identifying your own perspective on personhood is a fundamental prerequisite to being able to identify spiritual needs in your client. It is something we don't often take the time to do, but it is a very rich and rewarding experience to know yourself. There certainly is fundamental agreement in the nursing theoretical literature that the person is more than a body/mind, and nursing care is more than just meeting physical needs (Rogers, 1990; Levine, 1989; Neuman, 1982; Watson, 1979, 1985; Roy, 1984; King 1981; Parse, 1987; Fitzpatrick, 1983; Newman, 1989). Reading some of these theorists' perspectives of the person will help you to clarify your points of agreement and tension. The spiritual dimension is accepted by most nurse theorists, but located differently with varying levels of influence on the whole being. In some models the concept of spirituality is embedded, while in others it is a major concept of the nursing theory. Martsolf and Mickley (1998) provide an excellent precis that is a useful starting point for your reading. How you perceive the person will influence how you assess, prioritise and deliver your nursing practice.

To demonstrate the importance of identifying your personal perspective, I have clarified my own view of the person to demonstrate how this influences the way I enact my nursing practice within a nurse–client relationship. I see humans as personal, individual beings, created by God, in God's image, for a purpose; endowed with freedom to choose how they will live and the responsibility and self-awareness this freedom demands. The person is always living in relationship with self, other people, the environment and God (however the person interprets 'God'). Such a perspective means I perceive the client as having a unique God-given purpose. I have a responsibility to enhance the client's life choices and opportunities, so they can fulfil and maintain their sense of purpose. I seek to sustain the client's vital relationships to enhance their health and wellbeing. When I am expected to care for a client, we can both choose to be in the relationship at various levels. We may choose to meet at a 'deeper' personal level, or we may choose to remain 'distant'. This choice is influenced by many factors, some within my control and others beyond my control, but the consequences of our choice will affect us both. We all come to the nurse–client interface with our values in place. Identifying your values, beliefs and attitudes about the person helps to situate your practice, which in turn facilitates your ability to identify the client's perspective and thus meet their spiritual needs.

activity 1

These ten questions will begin to help you to be aware of your perspective of the person, and the values you embrace. Spend a little time reflecting on your position before undertaking each question.

1 Jot down ten values or beliefs you hold about personhood.
2 If you were asked to describe 'the real you', what would you say?
3 What gives your life a sense of meaning and purpose?
4 What are your life goals?
5 What are some of the personal values that have shaped your life goals?
6 How would you describe or define the human spirit?
7 Discuss the comment 'The body is just a vehicle for the spirit'.
8 Discuss this comment by Florence Nightingale '. . . they flit around like angels without hands among the patients and soothe their souls while they leave their bodies dirty and neglected' (quoted in Woodham-Smith, 1950, p. 109).

9 How do your relationships with other people shape the person you are?

10 Can you recount experiences with the environment that you might identify as spiritually meaningful?

To develop your self-awareness further, try some of the many excellent exercises included in Fish and Shelley (1988).

why should we bother assessing a person's spiritual needs?

Crisis and loss situations are the causal conditions of spiritual needs. Ageing can be marked by a series of losses which lead to challenges to the person's sense of meaning, purpose, hope, forgiveness, love, belonging, transcendence, and relationships with God, others and the environment; thus leading to spiritual needs (Stallwood and Stoll, 1975; Carson, 1989; Reed, 1992; van Loon, 1995). When these needs are attended to, they can add up to an improved quality of living for older people. The causal conditions for these spiritual needs include physical trauma, acute illness, terminal illness, loneliness and isolation, actual and/or perceived use and abuse of the person, imminent death and death (van Loon, 1995). These 'crises' present choice points that force new patterns of living (Newman, 1989). They often lead to 'loss' experiences, which may include loss of body parts or function, lifestyle, love, meaningful relationships, self-esteem and self worth, mental function, and loss of life itself. Let's just take a quick look at the key spiritual needs of people that lead to these loss experiences.

the need for meaning and purpose in life

Meaning and purpose are fundamental requisites for humans to achieve spiritual wellbeing (van Loon, 1995, p. 128). You cannot provide meaning for your client. Highfield and Cason (1983) point out that meaning is achieved through sociocultural influences and the formulation or adoption of a personal philosophy in life. Crisis can result in your client losing the 'will to live' as they no longer perceive a 'reason for living' (van Loon, 1995, p. 129). Religion may provide an organised and formalised framework with which the person can construct their life, providing the guiding principles to give expression to their sense of life's meaning and purpose. A quote from a nurse working with oncology clients illustrates how you, the nurse, can direct the focus of care to the spiritual dimension to maximise support for your client: '. . . her religion was all she had to hold together her threads of hope, so that was where I turned my attention' (ibid., p. 114). Australia's pluralist society provides a melting pot of diverse cultures, religions and philosophies from which clients derive their personally constructed meanings and purposes in life. Facilitating access to the person's philosophical frameworks and nurturing these structures becomes integral to meeting your client's spiritual needs.

the need for love and belonging

People need to love themselves to be able to give love and to receive love from others. Clients with major bodily dysfunction, who abuse themselves or have been victims of abuse, clients with mental illness and clients who have little family support, have particularly strong needs in this area (van Loon, 1995). These people feel unloved and have difficulty loving themselves, which greatly decreases their sense of wellbeing. Caring for these clients is time consuming, because it takes longer to establish a trusting and meaningful nurse–client relationship. Thus, time commitment should be factored into your decision to attend to their spiritual needs. The outcomes are less predictable and are often less positive, as it takes significant energy and skill to create the interpersonal relationship that can facilitate a positive outcome (ibid., p. 131). Your compassionate presence, genuine concern and empathy can help the client feel valued and less isolated. When you display these qualities, clients may comment that they no longer feel as if they are suffering alone and they may speak of feeling valued and worthwhile because they are accepted by the nurse (ibid., p. 130).

Many clients with religious beliefs additionally need to sustain a loving relationship with 'God'. This loving relationship can be greatly challenged when an older person is undergoing a series of crises and losses. Finding God in their suffering may be helpful and is best handled by pastoral care experts and clergy, as this area requires significant time to explore feelings and attitudes. Assessing your client's need must translate into some form of action to meet the need, which should include referral to people with the time and expertise in this domain of care.

the need for hope

Hope has two facets: one looks within to the transcending spirit, a relationship with 'God' and a hope in an afterlife; the second relates to hope for current experiences as the following example demonstrates. I observed a nurse giving an elderly man small tasks to do. The first day his goal was to wash his face; the next day, to do his hair; day three, to clean his teeth. Each day he saw he could do more for himself. The nurse gave gentle encouragement, and the client became more hopeful that he would be able to look after himself again. Hope gave the impetus to move forward (van Loon, 1995, p. 133). The way your client structures meaning in life usually leads to their source of hope. Hope cannot be provided, but only ignited from within. This is achieved by assisting your client to reframe their perspective and, if possible, providing the incentive to do so (ibid.).

the need for forgiveness

Reed (1992) discusses how some clients experience guilt, which causes great spiritual distress. Two common causes of guilt include unresolved conflict in human relationships and guilt over health status. The degree of guilt experienced depends on the history of the source of your client's guilt. This means your client may need extensive periods of counselling to reveal the source of their guilt before they are able to seek reconciliation. Referring your client to specialist nurses, pastoral care workers and other health professionals for counselling is generally the best way to meet this need. It is better not to start opening wounds of the past unless you have the time and skills to manage what you begin. As this nurse states, 'You rip the scab off a wound which has been festering for so long and then leave it raw and exposed. It is not right to do that' (van Loon, 1995, p. 137).

the need for a relationship with 'God' and transcendence of the spirit

Depending on how your client interprets their spiritual dimension, a need for a relationship with God may or may not be present (Fish and Shelley, 1988). It is the spirit within people that desires to bond with God. Such a metaphysical concept requires you to have thought through your own perspective with some clarity. The human spirit is concerned with a vertical relationship with God, and a horizontal relationship with the spirits of other humans (Carson, 1989; Piles, 1990). I would include a relationship with the environment as a third dimension to spiritual well-being (van Loon, 1995). The vertical relationship transcends earthly experiences. It is a 'call' from God, that requires a response from the person. The subsequent relationship between God and the person is based on faith and trust, and alters the client's ways of being, doing, living, thinking and reacting (ibid., p. 138). Meeting your client's needs will be based upon how overt their religious expression is and how dependent the client is on assistance to meet their needs. For some people, the relationship is intensely private and personal and they will not entertain the thought of third party involvement. Other clients will require your assistance in maintaining and nurturing these relationships through activities such as prayer, meditation, the arts, rituals and sacraments. The only certain way you have of knowing the client's position is to ask. Very few clients will openly ask for assistance in the spiritual and religious dimensions of care, yet very few will decline assistance when it is offered (van Loon, 1995). If you feel comfortable in this domain, it will facilitate open questioning and responding and lead to quality nurse–client interaction.

how should we assess a client's spiritual needs?

Your nursing assessment of spiritual needs is the first phase of the nursing process illustrated in Figure 4.1, which has steps similar those in the eight-stage problem solving model discussed in Chapter 1. This assessment involves three major factors: your client, the situation, and you the nurse. The assessment process is one of information gathering and interpreting. Whenever you interpret, you are always doing so through your own perspective. What you think you are seeing, you will assign meaning to from your own frame of reference. You may begin this assessment of the client's spiritual needs by anticipating (before contact with the client) what needs they may be likely to be experiencing. During initial comprehensive and ongoing assessment (which continues for the entire nursing process of spiritual care), you check the client's recognition of their needs and their responses to the care you have initiated (see Figure 4.1).

four types of assessment

The nursing process of spiritual care begins with your assessment of the client's spiritual needs using any of the following four pathways: cognitive assessment, assessment by observing, assessment by communicating verbally and assessment by written communication.

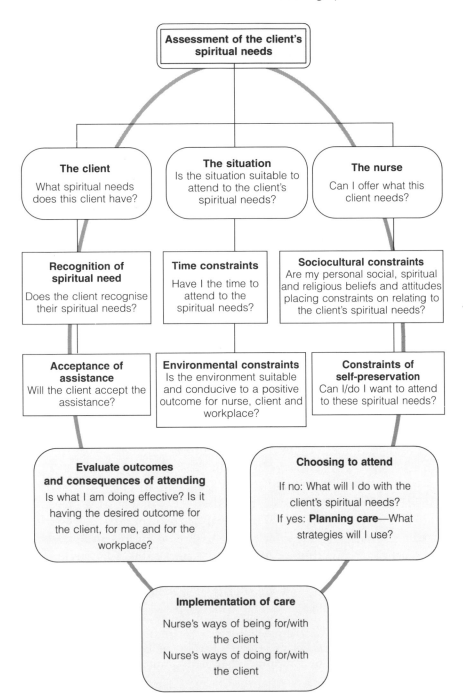

Figure 4.1: *The nursing process of spiritual care (© Antonia van Loon 1998)*

cognitive assessment

You will use your past nursing and life experience to anticipate your client's spiritual needs. An example would be anticipating the sense of dislocation and loss a client may be feeling on admission into a nursing home. You may pick up 'vibes' intuitively from your client (van Loon, 1995, p. 141), assuming potential needs of the client by reflecting and pondering on their situation. This is often described by nurses as 'sensing' a need.

assessment by observing

Assessment by observing your client's physical signs, behavioural cues, body language, their interactions with others and their immediate environment, will indicate the presence of spiritual needs.

assessment by communicating verbally

This involves communicating verbally during the client's formal oral history, verbal nursing 'hand-overs'; and informal conversation with the client, family, nurses and other health workers.

assessment by written communication

This involves using written communication such as nursing admission forms, and medical and nursing case notes. Formal assessments of spiritual needs may be of use in long-term care settings. Personal preference usually leads you to a preferred selection. I have listed a variety from the literature for your consideration. They include Stoll (1979), Paloutzian and Ellison (1982), Ellison (1983), Ellerhorst-Ryan (1988), Fish and Shelley (1988), Carson (1989), Westberg (1990) and Fitchett (1993). Carpenito (1983) published a guide to the North American Nursing Diagnosis (NANDA) that includes the diagnosis of spiritual distress. Carpenito's model of spiritual assessment uses five simple questions, which open the topic of spirituality up for further discussion and clarification. The questions tend to focus on the religious frameworks that bolster the client's spiritual dimension, but they are still a useful starting point to enter the subject of specific spiritual needs with clients. Carpenito's (1983, p. 452) questions are:

- Is religion or God important to you? If the answer is yes, to what religion do you belong? Or in what do you believe? If the answer is no, do you find a source of strength or meaning in another area?
- What effect do you expect your illness (hospitalisation) to have on your spiritual practices or beliefs?

- Are there any religious books (statues, medals, services, places) that are especially important to you?
- Do you have a special religious leader (priest, pastor, rabbi)?
- How can I help you maintain your spiritual strength during this illness (hospitalisation) (eg, contact a spiritual leader, provide privacy at special times, request reading materials)?

The main deficit in this model is its illness focus. Westberg and Westberg (1990, pp. 85–90) have developed a model which posits an alternative wellness focus, discovering how the person copes with life changes and how they nurture their relationship with God, others and themselves. All models are only as useful as the action that follows the assessment. It is not enough to ask the questions; you then have to do something with your findings.

Spiritual needs assessment may take any of four trajectories:

- assessment directly initiated by your client
- assessment indirectly initiated by your client
- assessment unilaterally initiated by the nurse before interaction with the client
- assessment unilaterally initiated by the nurse after interaction with the client.

assessment directly initiated by your client

This is the easiest trajectory for you the nurse, but the least commonly observed. Your client recognises they have needs. This does not imply they necessarily recognise these needs as spiritual, but that your client recognises they have needs in the area you would define as the spiritual dimension. Clients stimulate your awareness of their needs by directly requesting assistance from you. An example demonstrates: 'I knew he was religious because he had a photo of a guru around his neck. He wanted quiet time to meditate . . . so he asked me directly, if I could do something about it. He wanted to go for his tests in a relaxed state and he needed some peace and quiet to do his meditation' (van Loon, 1995, p. 164).

assessment indirectly initiated by your client

Your client may indirectly initiate a spiritual needs assessment, either unintentionally or deliberately, by means of behavioural and environmental cues and clues. After recognising their spiritual needs, your client may hint about their desire for assistance, as this example demonstrates:

'She had her religious objects on her table top and she clung to at least one, whenever she had anything done to her. I felt sure she wanted me to ask her about them so I did. She obviously wanted to share what was meaningful to her . . .' (van Loon, 1995, p. 165).

assessment initiated by the nurse before interaction with the client

In this trajectory you may perceive (in an almost intuitive and certainly immediate fashion) that your client has spiritual needs. This judgment is based in part on your previous experience and theoretical knowledge. You can then incorporate the needs into your client care assessment, designing strategies to attend to them in the care plan. Planning care in this trajectory usually occurs in your mind, so don't forget to document your assessment findings in the formal care plan and the case notes. You may choose to validate your assessment by clarifying the needs directly or indirectly with your client. If the needs are validated, this usually occurs at a later juncture in the caring trajectory. The personal and private nature of the spiritual dimension lead most nurses to approach needs clarification in an indirect manner—so indirect that the word 'spiritual' is rarely mentioned. It is easier to ask your client indirectly rather than asking them if they have any spiritual problems; a less direct assessment question usually gets a worthwhile response and is less threatening to them and to you. However, an unfortunate consequence of 'hiding' this assessment process is the fact that it is rarely documented. This lack of documentation leads to undervaluing of the impact spiritual care has on quality nursing care. As a result, it cannot be facilitated as it has not been costed within the formulae for funding care, because it is hidden in the ordinary actions of nursing and thus taken for granted.

assessment initiated by the nurse after interaction with the client

This form of assessment is the most common trajectory in use. It is often obfuscated, because it is situated within the realm of 'ordinary' nursing care as this nurse states: 'If you are around them long enough, you begin to know how they tick, and you soon know what their needs are, without always having to discuss and confirm it' (van Loon, 1995, p. 170).

Your client may or may not recognise their needs as spiritual and you may or may not validate the needs with your client. Sometimes your client does not recognise the need as spiritual, yet continues to provide you with unintentional cues. If this is the case, you might choose to attend to spiritual needs without ever discussing them with your client. Outcomes are just as satisfactory for your client, and many nurses comment that they feel more comfortable with this approach because it avoids embarrassment over what is considered to be personal and private. This nurse's comment illustrates: 'I am embarrassed to call them spiritual needs even though I know they are, because people might think I am a religious nut and I am not!' (van Loon, 1995, p. 170). Once again, don't forget to document your assessment findings and subsequent outcomes of care in the case notes.

Assessment is ongoing for the duration of your nurse–client relationship. You should ask yourself if the situation is appropriate to attend to any spiritual needs assessed. The flow charts in Figures 4.2 and 4.3 clearly demonstrate conceptually, the relationships and linkages of this assessment process when it is initiated by your client (Figure 4.2) and when it is initiated by you, the nurse (Figure 4.3). The trajectories follow distinct decision trails that are useful critical pathways to guide your decision making in the spiritual assessment process.

activity 2

For each of the following case studies, use the flow charts in Figures 4.2 and 4.3 to:

- Identify the potential and actual spiritual need(s) of the client.
- State the clues and cues you can pick up from the scenario.
- Identify which pathway your assessment might follow and state your rationale for choosing this pathway.
- List any constraints likely to affect your choice to attend to the identified needs.

Note: Some psychosocial needs have a deep impact on the spiritual wellbeing of the person and, as such, are identified as spiritual needs.

case study 1: Mr Z

Mr Z is a new resident at 'Blue Hills Home', a comprehensive residential care facility. He has multiple pathology that includes chronic lung disease, type 2 diabetes (non-insulin dependent diabetes mellitus), and mild heart failure. Mr Z, a widower, migrated to Australia in 1958 from Italy and has one son living in Melbourne and no family living close by.

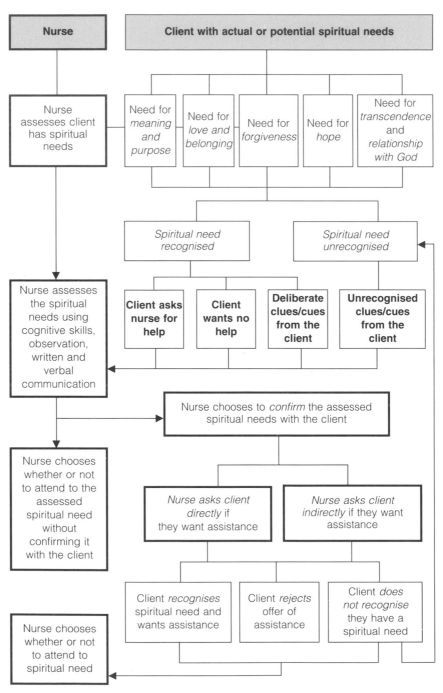

Figure 4.2: *Client initiated assessment of spiritual needs (© Antonia van Loon 1998)*

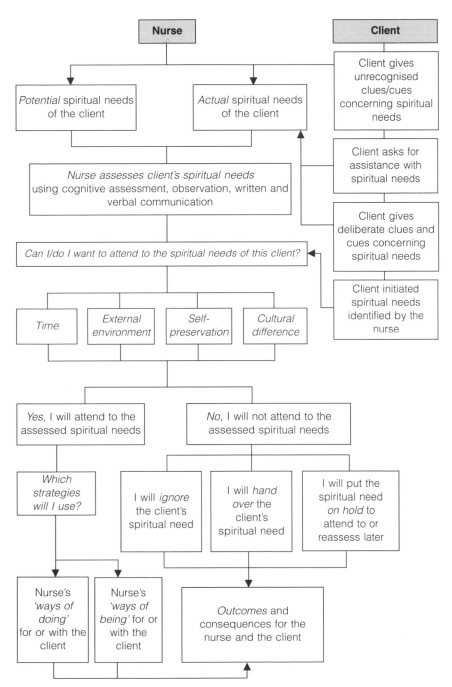

Figure 4.3: *Nurse initiated assessment of spiritual needs* (© *Antonia van Loon 1998*)

Mr Z smoked one packet of cigarettes a day for 40 years, a fact his son finds disgusting. Mr Z is a member of the Roman Catholic Church and he attended mass each week before coming to Blue Hills. He wears a gold crucifix around his neck and keeps his rosary beads on his locker top.

You are the nurse coming on night duty. On one of your rounds you find Mr Z awake, sitting upright with some mild nocturnal dyspnoea. He is anxious and restless, and is clinging to his rosary beads. You settle his shortness of breath with a bronchodilator but he is still visibly upset and anxious.

case study 2: Mrs S

You are the home visiting nurse of Mrs S, who lives on her own in a two-bedroom unit. She has just returned home from a visit interstate to see her daughter and grandchildren. Mrs S tells you her daughter recently separated from her husband and is struggling to cope with work and the children. She misses her daughter and grandchildren and is disappointed she can't be there to help her daughter out more with the care of the children.

She comments that her daughter was very upset and the children did not want to see her leave. Mrs S states, 'I felt so guilty leaving them. I can't be there for the kids when they need me . . .'. She goes on to discuss how lonely she feels and that she just can't cope any more with all the pressures of the family. She says, 'I can't understand why God allows all this suffering to happen to us'.

case study 3: Mr B

Mr B was an elder and lay preacher in his church for many years. He now has carcinoma of the prostate and is receiving end-stage palliative care from you in his home. He has a very supportive family and friends from his faith community who provide ongoing support for the family by way of meals, regular visits and religious support. One evening while you are sponging Mr B, he confides in you that he thinks God has left him and that he is '. . . really scared of dying' but he doesn't dare to tell anyone from his church for fear that they will think him weak.

case study 4: Miss W

Miss W is a fit and healthy older woman who comes to your health clinic to get some dietary information. During your discussion, she comments about a photograph of a peaceful scene that you have on your wall. 'I used to enjoy photography', she says, 'but not any more. I can't see properly any more. I can't even hold the camera still now. I don't like this getting older . . . might as well be dead really . . . I just seem to be losing one thing I love, after another . . .'.

when should we attend to the assessed spiritual needs?

Your decision to attend will be based on your needs assessment, intervening conditions and your ability to achieve a positive outcome for you (the nurse) and your client. You may feel intuitively matched to a client's needs, or you may work this out through a process of deductive thinking and inductive reasoning. You will have to decide whether to attend to the needs, to reassess and/or attend to them later, to hand over the needs, or to ignore the spiritual needs altogether.

The correct time to assess and attend to spiritual needs depends on your ability to control the following intervening conditions. These include: environmental, personal, time and cultural considerations. You must consider whether you need a quiet, private place to ensure client confidentiality. You must consider your own need to preserve yourself. You should ask yourself, 'Do I have the personal desire, energy, ability and knowledge to assist this client?'. Your philosophical worldview of people and your perception of your nursing role will influence this decision. The availability of time to attend to the client's spiritual needs will influence your choice to attend. Time considerations are affected by the assessed depth and severity of your client's needs, your current workload and that of the workplace, the ability of other nursing team members to support your endeavour, your role within the team, your orientation to nursing tasks, and the time you and your client have available to meet the assessed spiritual needs.

There are also cultural variables that will affect your choice to attend to spiritual needs. Australian societal norms concerning the personal and private nature of spirituality and religion stop many nurses from discussing this dimension of care with the client. You will probably find it easier to attend to the needs of clients who are from a similar cultural, philosophical and spiritual orientation as yourself. However, you are also responsible for meeting the spiritual needs of clients from different cultures and religions. The subculture of your workplace will also influence your choice to attend. This will include peer reactions, hospital philosophy, and the guidelines and models of nursing practice in use. After assessing these conditions, you will decide whether or not to attend to the spiritual needs. If you choose not to attend yourself, you will have to decide what to do with the assessed spiritual need. This usually involves either reassessing and/or attending to the need later, handing over the need to another professional, or choosing to ignore the need altogether. If you chose to attend, you will have to decide which strategy you will use to deal with the spiritual needs. These strategies can be broadly categorised into 'ways of doing' and 'ways of being'.

strategies for dealing with spiritual needs

'ways of doing' to meet a client's spiritual needs

You can use a variety of 'ways of doing' with, or for, the client to ameliorate their spiritual needs. The 'doing' activities often include purposeful additions to the normal daily tasks and routines that take place within the ordinary nurse–client relationship. These include creating an appropriate environment; enlisting the support of other people, including family, friends and other professionals; encouraging and promoting the movement of the client towards independence; and facilitating the client's religious beliefs and practices.

Environmental changes may be made to nurture and sustain the person's inner peace. These include reducing unnecessary noise and creating privacy and seclusion, as required. You can provide music, literature, art works, photographs and religious symbols as means of creating an environment conducive to reflection, meditation and the provision of temporary release.

Enlist the support of other people who can help the person re-establish spiritual wellbeing. These may include family, friends, support groups, community agencies, religious experts and other health professionals with skills to assist the client with their needs. The family group is, for most people, one of the major influences in the formulation of values and beliefs that sustain the spiritual dimension.

You can promote independence as a means of attending to spiritual needs by encouraging and promoting self-care, mobility, creative expression and purposeful activity. Promoting independence is one method of rekindling hope and a sense of purpose in life. Maintaining independence has been shown to lead to motivation, empowerment, self-worth and personal value, which enhance spiritual wellbeing (van Loon, 1995, p. 230).

You can facilitate the client's ability to draw on their religious beliefs and practices such as festivals, rituals, meditative opportunities, prayer and religious symbols; and provide opportunities for worship and praise. For many clients, their religion provides the framework upon which they have built their hope, meaning and purpose in life.

'ways of being' to meet a client's spiritual needs

During these 'doing' activities, you can use yourself therapeutically through various 'ways of being' which include dialogue with the client, your compassionate presence, and using various forms of connecting with the client. Dialogue with the client involves you informing, sharing, paraphrasing, questioning, confronting, reassuring, mediating, joking and planning. You use yourself by offering your compassionate presence to the client by being available, listening attentively, sitting with the client, anticipating the client's needs, and being there for the duration of the experience. This involves a special, more intimate nurse–client relationship than is usually the case, as this nurse's comments suggest: 'I am giving something of myself . . . I feel O.K. about being in their personal space and they have done the same . . . it is almost sacred . . . you can't get into it without putting yourself on the line' (van Loon, 1995, p. 212).

There is a connection of spirits that occurs through caring touch (Stiles, 1990). The elderly, in particular, need this caring touch to make them feel secure and cared for. Older people will often reach out to touch you as you pass by, and hang onto you when they are touched, not wanting to let go. It can make you feel uncomfortable and exposed, but the caring physical touch is a very close correlate to spiritual connection. As this nurse comments: 'It is raw humanity, encountering a person who is exposed and exposing yourself . . . who you really are . . . you cannot get a closer, more intimate, or a more vulnerable moment in nursing' (van Loon, 1995, p. 212).

Connecting with clients who are dying is again a special way of attending to the spiritual needs of this special group of people. The following comment made by an oncology nurse illustrates this point: 'We assist the passage of the dying person's spirit, allowing the spirit to travel on to its destination—home' (van Loon, 1995, p. 213).

the context of spiritual care: the nurse–client relationship

A 'special' nurse–client relationship is a consequence of as well as a pre-condition for assessment and attending to spiritual needs of the person.

This special relationship takes place within your 'ordinary' nurse–client alliance. Respect and genuine concern are essential prerequisites for positive outcomes. A special nurse–client relationship is fostered if you accept, value and respect your client, demonstrating empathy and sympathy for them and their situation in a non-judgmental and non-threatening manner.

evaluating consequences and outcomes of spiritual care

This is the last step in the process of spiritual care, where you should evaluate the outcomes of your care for you the nurse, your client and the workplace. Van Loon (1995, pp. 247–8) notes that outcomes for the client of this special nurse–client relationship include reduced anxiety, acceptance of their situation, empowerment, and feeling enabled, secure and comforted. You, the nurse, and your client can experience enhanced spiritual wellbeing and healing if your ability and your client's spiritual needs are matched. Both nurses and clients express feeling privileged, worthwhile, valued, respected, satisfied and uplifted.

Van Loon (1995, pp. 248–51) goes on to report that negative outcomes are possible when the client's needs and the nurse's ability are mismatched, or the intervening conditions are unable to be controlled. If the nurse's ability and client's spiritual needs are mismatched, both nurse and client express feeling trapped, stressed, confronted, used, dissatisfied, frustrated, fatigued, drained and burnt out. Therefore it is imperative that you decide whether the assistance you are offering is effective, accepted and desirable for all involved. This evaluation will affect the ongoing cycle of assessment, planning, implementation and evaluation of the nursing process of spiritual care, which is presented graphically in Figure 4.1.

conclusion

In this chapter I have introduced you to the concepts of spirituality, spiritual wellbeing, spiritual needs and spiritual care. I have discussed the key spiritual needs that most nurses are likely to encounter when caring for older people. These spiritual needs include the need for meaning and purpose in life, for love and belonging, hope, forgiveness, a relationship with God and transcendence of the human spirit. I have demonstrated the process of assessment of spiritual needs within the nursing process and provided two critical pathways to assist the decision-making process pertaining to assessment of spiritual needs and subsequent spiritual care. Ultimately, assessing spiritual needs requires some insight into your own beliefs and philosophical perspective and a willingness to identify these deeper needs in others. It involves a therapeutic use of self within the nurse–client relationship, which places both parties in a vulnerable position. Further, it requires a commitment to action when you have assessed these needs. This can be decided by evaluating several intervening conditions to spiritual care. I firmly believe that caring for your client's spiritual needs is what creates healing of the whole person, even when a cure is no longer a possibility. Spiritual care contributes to quality care of the whole person.

study questions

1   What are your personal definitions of spirituality, spiritual wellbeing, spiritual needs and spiritual care of the older person?
2   Think of a time when you felt you gave spiritual care and then answer the following questions:
    a   How did you know you gave spiritual care?
    b   What assessment process did you use?
    c   Try to retrace the decision on the flow charts and see if you can identify what facilitated your assessment process and your subsequent care.
3   What hinders your ability to provide spiritual care?
4   Identify three ways you can remove, or mitigate these obstacles.

references

Barker, E. R. D. (1989), 'Being whole: Spiritual wellbeing in Appalachian women a phenomenological study', Unpublished PhD dissertation, University of Texas, Austin, Texas.

Burkhardt, M. A. (1993), 'Characteristics of spirituality in the lives of women in a rural Appalachian community', *Journal of Transcultural Nursing*, Winter, 4(2), pp. 12–18.

Burns, P. G. (1989), 'The experience of spirituality in the well adult: A phenomenological study', Unpublished PhD dissertation, Texas Woman's University, Texas.

Carpenito, L. J. (1983), *Nursing Diagnosis: Application to Clinical Practice*, J. B. Lippincott Co, Philadelphia.

Carson, V. B. (1989), *Spiritual Dimensions of Nursing Practice*, W. B. Saunders, Philadelphia.

Conrad, N. L. (1985), 'Spiritual support for the dying', *Nursing Clinics of North America*, 24(2), pp. 415–26.

Dugan, D. O. (1987/88), 'Essays in the art of caring: The human spirit in stress management', *Nursing Forum*, XX111 (3), pp. 08–117.

Ellerhorst-Ryan, J. (1988), *Instruments for Clinical Nursing Research*, Appleton & Lange, Norwalk, Connecticut, p. 142.

Ellison, C. W. (1983), 'Spiritual wellbeing: Conceptualisation and measurement', *Journal of Psychology and Theology*, 11, pp. 330–40.

Emblen, J. D. (1992), 'Religion and spirituality defined according to current use in the nursing literature', *Journal of Professional Nursing*, Jan/Feb, 8(1), pp. 41–7.

Fish, S. and Shelly J. A. (1988), *Spiritual Care: The Nurse's Role*, 3rd edn, Intervarsity Press, Downers Grove, Illinois.

Fitchett, G. (1993), *Assessing Spiritual Needs: A Guide for Care Givers*, Augsburg Fortress, Minneapolis.

Fitzpatrick, J. J. (1983), 'A life perspective rhythm model' in J. J. Fitzpatrick and A. L. Whall (eds), *Conceptual Models of Nursing: Analysis and Applications*, 1st edn, M. D. Bowie, Robert, J. Brady, USA, pp. 295–302.

Highfield, M. F. and Cason, C. (1983), 'Spiritual needs of patients: Are they recognised?', *Cancer Nursing*, 6(3), pp. 187–92.

King, I. M. (1981), *A Theory for Nursing: Systems, Concepts, Process*, John Wiley & Sons, New York.

Levine, M. E. (1971), 'Holistic nursing', *Nursing Clinics of North America*, 6, pp. 253–64.

Levine, M. E. (1989), 'The four conservation principles: Twenty years later', in J. Riehl-Sisca (ed.), *Conceptual Models for Nursing Practice*, 3rd edn, Appleton Century Crofts, Norwalk, Connecticut, pp. 325–37.

Martsolf, D. S. and Mickley, J. R. (1998), 'The concept of spirituality in nursing theories: Differing world-views and extent of focus', *Journal of Advanced Nursing*, 27(2), pp. 294–303.

Neuman, B. (1982), *The Neuman Systems Model: Application to Nursing Education and Practice*, Appleton Century Crofts, Norwalk, Connecticut.

Newman, M. A. (1986), *Health as Expanding Consciousness*, C. V. Mosby, St Louis, Missouri.

Newman, M. A. (1989), 'The spirit of nursing', *Holistic Nursing Practice*, 3(3), pp. 1–6.

Paloutzian, R. and Ellison, C. (1982), 'Loneliness, spiritual wellbeing and quality of life' in L. A. Peplau and D. Perlman (eds), *Loneliness: A Sourcebook of Current Theory, Research and Therapy*, Wiley Interscience, New York.

Parse, R. R. (1987), 'Parse's man-living-health theory' in R. R. Parse (ed.), *Nursing Science: Major Paradigms, Theories and Critiques*, Saunders, Philadelphia, pp. 181–204.

Piles, C. L. (1990), 'Providing spiritual care', *Nurse Educator*, 15(1), pp. 36–41.

Reed, P. G. (1992), 'An emerging paradigm for the investigation of spirituality in nursing', *Research in Nursing and Health*, 15(5), pp. 349–57.

Rogers, M. E. (1970), *An Introduction to the Theoretical Basis of Nursing*, F. A. Davis, Philadelphia.

Rogers, M. E. (1990), 'Nursing science of unitary irreducible human beings: Update 1990' in E. A. Barrett (ed.), *Visions of Science Based Nursing*, National League of Nursing, New York.

Roy, C. Sr. (1984), *Introduction to Nursing: An Adaptation Model*, 2nd edn, Prentice Hall, Englewood Cliffs, New Jersey.

Stallwood, J. and Stoll R. (1975), 'Spiritual dimension of nursing practice' in I. L. Beland and J. Y. Passos (eds), *Clinical Nursing*, 3rd edn, Macmillan, New York.

Stiles, M. K. (1990), 'The shining stranger: Nurse–family spiritual relationship', *Cancer Nursing*, 13(4), pp. 235–45.

Stoll, R. (1979), 'Guidelines for spiritual assessment', *American Journal of Nursing*, 79(9), pp. 1574–7.

van Loon, A. M. (1995), 'What constitutes caring of the human spirit in nursing?', Unpublished MN (research) dissertation, Flinders University of South Australia, Adelaide.

Watson, J. (1979), *Nursing: The Philosophy and Science of Caring*, Little Brown, Boston.

Watson, J. (1985), *Nursing: Human Science and Human Care*, Appleton-Century-Croft, Norwalk, Connecticut.

Westberg, G. E. and Westberg McNamara, J. (1990), *The Parish Nurse: Providing a Minister of Health for your Congregation*, Augsburg Fortress, Minneapolis.

Woodham-Smith, C. (1950), *Florence Nightingale*, The Reprint Society, London.

Zerwekh, J. (1993), 'Transcending life: The practice wisdom of nursing hospice experts', *American Journal of Hospice and Palliative Care*, 10(5), pp. 26–31.

chapter 5

social and lifestyle assessment

Elery Hamilton Smith

chapter summary

The chapter opens with a brief review of the lifestyle concept and its importance in aged care. The assessment process is outlined, and then illustrated by documenting the lifestyle assessment of a fictitious Mr Jensen. Examples of assessment instruments are illustrated.

objectives

After reading and reflecting on this chapter, you will:

- be aware of the importance of understanding individual lifestyles
- understand the need to assess lifestyle requirements through life-span assessment
- be able to effectively use methods for assessing lifestyle requirements.

introduction

At the very simplest level, lifestyle has been defined as the whole range of things we do each week. This is, however, nothing more than a simple description and does not help us to apply the idea in everyday professional practice. There are a range of ways of thinking about lifestyle (Veal, 1993), but for present purposes, a particularly useful way of considering it (based largely in the ideas of the sociologist Max Weber) is that it represents the sum total of our claims to social status. The way we express these claims may vary according to the roles in which we find ourselves at a given point in time. At the one time, you may be a casually employed registered nurse, a spouse and parent, a member of a local church, and president of the local garden club, each of which demands a specific and often very different set of assumptions, beliefs, actions and relationships. But in our integration of them, so we summarise our roles and define our personal lifestyle. It further establishes our own self-image. This in turn enables others to define us, see us as one of a social group, and differentiate us from people who have a different lifestyle. Lifestyle is particularly useful in thinking about older people, as their wellbeing and happiness depends very largely upon the extent to which they can preserve a positive sense of social status.

When we think about a dependent older person in either family or residential care, the first and most obvious aspect of their lifestyle is that it is all to often constrained to a very narrow and low-status role: that of being a dependent older person in care. Florida Scott-Maxwell (1968, p. 91) expressed it poignantly:

> . . . Being ill in a nursing home became my next task, a sombre dance in which I knew some of the steps. I must conform. I must be correct. I must be meek, obedient and grateful, on no account must I be surprising.

This is clearly a demeaning and malignant situation. It challenges those responsible for care to preserve the individuality of those for whom they care and to treat them as total people with every respect and dignity. Such an approach demands the fullest possible understanding of each individual—hence this chapter.

why assess previous lifestyle?

Clearly, the lifestyle of the person in care is shaped largely by the routines and relationships that prevail within the care situation. Carers can optimise or drastically reduce the independence and freedom of those for whom they care, and they can provide the opportunity for a high level of continuing satisfaction and joy or for a life of frustration and boredom.

Good care demands that carers understand each person for whom they are caring. The resident should not be cared for in some mechanistic and uniform way imposed by the care establishment, as Scott-Maxwell's comment implies. Rather, the resident should be seen as a person in the fullest sense of that word, and quality care must be a response to their unique personality and needs. Even the simplest care protocol, such as the way in which an individual is addressed (eg, formally as Mrs Brown, informally as Elizabeth, or intimately with a family nickname) should be as the resident wishes. It may even be that the resident will have different expectations from different members of the care staff (eg, being Elizabeth to the Director, but Mrs Brown to the care staff).

Even more importantly, the relationship between lifestyle and wellness is so profound that consideration of health from a purely clinical perspective cannot be complete or even adequate. Making competent recommendations and decisions to safeguard the wellbeing of any individual must take lifestyle options and choices into account. To take only one aspect of lifestyle as an example, the maintenance of friendship networks, contributes at least as much to health as giving up smoking, and can be demonstrated in terms of ensuring longer life, a lower rate of infection or illness and more effective recovery from illness or trauma (House et al., 1988).

We have also discovered from recent research on dementia (Garratt and Hamilton-Smith, 1995; Kitwood, 1997) that even the particular way in which dementia expresses itself through a person's behaviour is largely shaped by their personal history. Certainly, we can only begin to understand that behaviour if we know their cultural and personal history. Then, maintenance of an appropriate lifestyle for each individual greatly reduces and often eliminates the so-called disordered behaviour that used to be accepted as an inevitable component of dementia.

Determination of what is appropriate rests upon the assessment of the person's cultural background and personal history. Indeed, progressive lifestyle-based care strategies can provide not only a happy and satisfying life for the individual with a dementing illness, but may even enable them to maintain a range of life skills and so continue much of their previous life pattern. This approach to care also enables people with dementia to not only live a happy and relatively stress-free life, but as a result, they suffer much lower levels of infection or other illness. This is readily explained by extrapolation from research on the relationship between levels of stress and the functioning of the immune system. So, the evidence from new understandings of dementia provides dramatic support for the remarkable importance of lifestyle in assessment and care for all people.

In summary, ageing people in care at any level can only live a happy and satisfying life if they have the opportunity for a personally appropriate lifestyle, and they can only maintain their optimal physical and emotional wellbeing if they have such a lifestyle.

methods of lifestyle assessment

Given current program constraints, assessment will often be carried out by interview in a professional space rather than the ageing person's own space. To compound this problem, the interview may well be time-limited and hence superficial. This chapter therefore responds by spelling out both optimal and minimal strategies. To commence, we need to lay down some basic principles that should underlie social assessment:

- Social assessment should be both comprehensive and detailed; that is, it should show both breadth and depth.
- It should take the total life span into account, as many of the key events that shaped lifestyle may have occurred many years ago, and we will only really understand, and be able to respond positively, to another person's lifestyle if we understand the forces which that person sees as having shaped it.
- Social assessment should be based primarily in the person's own perception and understanding of their life, even though this may be at variance with other evidence (eg, from their children).
- Other available evidence, including perceptions and understandings from other family members, should, however, be recorded as well, as it provides very important collateral data.

• Interview and other records must be seen as the property of the resident or his or her guardians, and therefore available to them at any time.

Formal assessment interviewing may take place prior to, during or shortly after intake to care; it may (and probably should) involve not only the individual concerned, but their family and even friends and neighbours. But the formal interview will inevitably be incomplete and further information will emerge informally over successive months. If this is judged to be of sufficient importance to be recorded, permission should be sought to do so. Any such records should always identify the source of information, and should always be open to the person concerned and their family or guardian.

An interview carried out in the person's own home will have more value, partly because the person being interviewed will be more comfortable and find it easier to talk openly. They will also be likely to show photographs or other artefacts that illustrate their story. Then the interviewer will have the opportunity of seeing the person in their own environment, which in turn will prompt questions and focus the interview more effectively. The very nature of the home setting and the visible artefacts also demonstrate aspects of lifestyle in a very explicit way, and so complement and expand upon the spoken story.

Other sources may be valuable. Reviewing family photographs with the family, reading a diary or asking the person concerned (providing they are able to do so) to write their life story are all potentially valuable. Kelleher (1993) provides an excellent guide to the use of this kind of information. Each program or establishment should develop its own protocols for social and lifestyle assessment, and Table 5.1 provides a guideline to the range of potential opportunities.

Social assessment should progressively cover the person's normal daily routine, their normal weekly pattern in the last several years prior to admission, and the story of their lifespan. These are deliberately placed in this order—it will be easier for people to deal with the immediate situation, and then the earlier background will progressively emerge. Each of these three aspects is discussed below, together with examples to guide development of the necessary documentation.

daily routines

Firstly, it is necessary to examine the normal daily routine, and any special variations throughout the normal week. Any specific program or

Table 5.1: *Potential protocols for social and lifestyle assessment*

Timing	Optimal program with contact possible before admission to program or establishment	Minimal program with no contact possible before admission
One to six months prior to admission	1 Formal assessment interview, preferably at home 2 Photographic record of home 3 Invite to show family photographs or other similar materials 4 If practical, invite person to compile their own biography	–
At time of admission	Update interview and orientation to program or establishment	1 Formal assessment interview 2 Invite family to make photographs or other materials available
Following admission	1 Continue to build data from informal contacts with family and other visitors, and continuing relationship with resident 2 Invite family to permit, or help, in developing photographic record of the care experience 3 Document ways in which social and lifestyle assessment facilitates care planning and management	Continue to update data, as possible, through contact with resident, family and other visitors

establishment will doubtless have their own schedules to guide or direct interviewing and other data gathering. However, Figure 5.1 depicts a useful format for collecting and recording this information. These outlines are not intended as a structure for interviewing; in general, inter-

Normal daily routine	
Time	
6.00 am	
7.00 am	
8.00 am	Gets up, coffee, showers, dresses, breakfast, listens to news (in that order)
9.00 am	Reads paper
10.00 am	Gardens, or walks down to local park and shops
11.00 am	
12.00 pm	
1.00 pm	Lunch, generally at home
2.00 pm	Reads, or sometimes has a nap
3.00 pm	
4.00 pm	Visits or is visited by friends, or meets at local coffee shop
5.00 pm	
6.00 pm	Watches TV news
6.30 pm	Dinner
7.30 pm	TV
9.00 pm	Bed, unless special program on TV
10.00 pm	
11.00 pm	
12.00 am	
Include: Getting up, bedtime Showering All meals Cups of tea, etc. All other regular events (exercise, housework, etc)	

Daily variations	
Monday	
Tuesday	Often a night at the theatre or cinema
Wednesday	
Thursday	
Friday	
Saturday	May visit or go on an outing with friends
Sunday	
Include: Household chores Regular visits or outings	

Figure 5.1: *The daily routine*

viewing should be as informal and free-flowing as possible to help the older person feel at ease. With forms of this kind, the data can be recorded as it emerges and specific prompts or questions used to fill any gaps.

This is a relatively simple component of the assessment, and simply provides the information that should be used in constructing the daily routine aspects of the care plan. It is only in the next step that real lifestyle characterisation starts to emerge. Here the interview has to step back from simple routines and commence an examination of what really matters to the individual.

We will look at the information from a hypothetical person, Mr Jensen, to give a case study example of the interview process. In introducing Mr Jensen, let's imagine that he has enquired about entering a hostel, largely as a result of pressure from his brother and an appointment made for him by his brother. He has been assessed to ascertain whether this is an appropriate step to take. The social assessment alone indicates that his brother may be over-concerned, and that on the whole, he is able to manage his own life. However, for other reasons, it has been decided that he should be offered a place. Thus, the example here is a pre-entry assessment of a man who has lived a very narrowly focused life.

the normal lifestyle

The normal pattern of life over the few years immediately prior to assessment must next be explored. This life pattern will inevitably be reconstructed by admission to a care program, but an understanding of it provides the basis upon which we can best provide for that reconstruction. Basic to a satisfactory assessment at this level are the trends and changes that are in process. No person remains static, and a truly sympathetic care program needs to not only recognise these trends, but to consider which should be maintained and which might be changed in a more positive direction.

The interview should endeavour to elucidate which components of life are the most important to the person concerned, and to make a provisional assessment of which directions might best be emphasised for the future. In this part of the interview, a sensitive assessment of the person's home environment can greatly add to and strengthen the overall picture.

Again, most establishments will have a procedure in place. Table 5.2

Table 5.2: *Normal lifestyle over the last few years*

Item	Details	Trends and recent changes
Housing (eg, character of home, preferred rooms, favourite furniture, garden)	Apartment with living room, bedroom, kitchenette and bathroom. Very small but lovely garden bed	–
Outings and community activities Linkages with friendships, leisure interests, church, etc	No involvement with formal organisations but see below	–
Friendships Importance, patterns of interaction	Has a network of close friends who visit him regularly, or whom he visits. They also share outings	–
Family relations Patterns of interaction and dependence/ independence	His only family contact is sporadic and with a brother who feels concerned about him	Brother wants him to enter hostel care as he believes Mr Jensen is no longer able to care properly for himself
Meals Who prepares, preferences, timing, snacks between meals	Cooks for himself—is particular about quality of his food	It seems that he is cooking less, and increasingly relying on odd snacks of take-away food, or forgetting to eat at all
Work Paid or unpaid, home, garden	Keeps apartment and garden in immaculate condition	Seems to be less particular than previously, apartment and garden somewhat untidy
Interests Leisure activities, hobbies, etc	Gardening, reading, being with friends	–
Beliefs and values Spirituality, personal relationships, behaviour, etc	Avowed agnostic, relates well to all friends and others and enjoys doing so, conventional but sociable	–
Memories, satisfactions, regrets	Seems quite centred upon theatre, very happy career with high satisfaction, comfortable with retirement	Has commented that his career did not leave time for family life and as friends die, feels increasingly lonely
Other	Great sense of humour; but sometimes sarcastic, which may upset other people	–

simply provides an example of the kind of format that might be used for data gathering.

documenting the life span

This is the most difficult component of the assessment and may be time-consuming, but it is vital to a full understanding of the person. In the case of those with dementia (or who move into dementia at a later date), it is absolutely essential. Many of the issues and concerns that emerge during dementia have their bases back in the earlier life of the person, and so the response to them must be also based in that earlier experience. There is much individual variation in life history. The most useful way to get a first overview is to commence with a chart similar to that shown in Figure 5.2 with only the first column completed, showing annual dates for at least the previous 75 years—longer if the interview occurs at a greater age. Commence (prior to interview, if possible) by filling in the person's age in the second column. This provides two kinds of markers against which events can be identified and located; some people will recall things in terms of dates and some in terms of their age, but most people will find the two together make it easier. Then track the key events: schooling, marriage, birth of children, war service, housing moves, employment, separation or divorce, deaths of family members and the like. This is still only a framework, but it is now detailed enough that you can discuss what was important at each period of the respondent's life.

Then in summarising, again try to identify the most important continuing and long-term themes and most memorable successes in the person's life. These are the kind of events that generate not only great pleasure, but that make a major contribution to the individual's sense of identity and self-image.

Interestingly, if a life history of this kind is compiled prior to the individual developing dementia, it may well demand some progressive updating as the memories that emerge in dementia may be about deeply felt events and emotions that were too painful or embarrassing to discuss previously.

conclusion

The three forms suggested here for the recording of assessment interviews or visits also provide a useful format for the final summary of each

Date	Age	Key events	Other important memories
		High school	Good student, loved English literature, happy
1944	17	Left school	Worked in parents' shop, but in repertory theatre at night
1945	18		Part-time and irregular work in theatre
1946	19		First radio drama experience with ABC
1947	20		
1948	21		
1949	22		First professional lead role in theatre
1950	23		
1951	24	Moved to London	Regular professional roles
1952	25		
1953	26		
1954	27		Joined Old Vic company
1955	28		
1956	29		
1957	30		Appeared in Royal Command performance
1958	31	Returned to Australia	
A diversity of roles in both theatre and radio drama			
1990	63		
1991	64		Grandfather role in radio serial
1992	65		
1993	66		
1994	67	Retirement	Radio serial ended—disappointed so decided to retire
1995	68		Holiday in Britain; bought present apartment
1996	69		
1997	70		

Figure 5.2: *An example of a life-span chart (part only) as both an interviewing aid and a pro forma for recording*

of the three windows upon lifestyle. But the assessment might also be summarised in a paragraph that brings together what appear to be the key aspects of the individual's preferred lifestyle and provides basic information to care staff. For instance:

Mr Jensen is a former professional actor, who has great pride in his profession and his personal achievements. He enjoys reminiscing about his experiences in both theatre and radio, and making comments upon, or relating jokes about, his former colleagues. He takes great pride in his personal appearance, but prefers informality in communication with other people. He is relatively independent and likes spending time on his own, but at the same time, he always enjoys informal gatherings with old friends, often over a late afternoon drink. Another important interest is his small garden, and his joy in having vases of flowers in his apartment. He never married, yet enjoys the company of, and talking with, women. His pattern of eating is irregular, and he may miss a meal, but then make up for it with occasional snacks.

The next step in documenting Mr Jensen's care should be a care plan or daily living plan (Garratt and Hamilton-Smith, 1995, pp. 141–51). This will clearly have to respond to his sociability, continuation of his friendship networks, interest in gardening and maintenance of his independence and self-reliance for as long as possible.

study questions

1   Given the limitations of time, what guidelines would you set for your own practice in order to ensure both depth and breadth of social assessment?
2   Assume a situation where there are significant disagreements between the story as told by the person who is the subject of a social assessment and their daughter. Obviously both stories should be recorded, but on what principles would you decide which elements of the two stories should be used in care planning?
3   Given what you know of Mr Jensen's story, what are the key aspects of his social history that should be used?

references

Garratt, S. and Hamilton-Smith, E. (eds) (1995), *Rethinking Dementia: An Australian Approach*, Ausmed Publications, Melbourne.
House, J. S., Landis, K. R. and Umberson, D. (1988), 'Social relationships and health', *Science*, 241, pp. 540–5.
Kellehear, A. (1993), *The Unobtrusive Researcher: A Guide to Methods*, Allen & Unwin, Sydney.

Kitwood, T. (1997), *Dementia Reconsidered: The Person Comes First*, Open University Press, Buckingham, UK.

Scott-Maxwell, F. (1968), *The Measure of My Days*, Knopf, New York.

Veal, A. J. (1993), 'The concept of lifestyle: A review', *Leisure Studies*, 12(4), pp. 233–52.

assessment for
clinical practice

assessing mental health

Michael Hazelton

chapter summary

This chapter outlines the components of a comprehensive mental health assessment for an older person in any health care setting. The theoretical and conceptual bases to mental health assessment and an overview of the most common mental disorders found in older people is provided. The chapter concludes with a brief discussion on the relationship between mental health assessment and evaluation of mental health outcomes, from the perspective of evidence-based practice.

objectives

After reading and reflecting on this chapter, you will:

- be able to demonstrate an understanding of mental health problems experienced by older people
- be able to question the therapeutic pessimism commonly associated with older people with mental problems and disorders
- have an understanding of the requirements to conduct mental health assessment
- have the capability to undertake a comprehensive mental health assessment of an older person.

introduction

While the proposition that mental health and physical health are inseparable might seem obvious, the history of health care in countries such as Australia indicates that, until recently, mental health has generally been isolated from mainstream health services and assigned low priority. In recent decades the neglect of mental health services has at last begun to be addressed by policy makers. Nowadays, mental health services are integrated into mainstream health services and the provision of comprehensive, community-based, consumer-oriented mental health services has become a policy priority (Australian Health Ministers, 1998).

While these developments have had a major impact in some parts of our health care system, elsewhere there have been delays. The provision of high quality mental health care for the older person has been one such area of delayed development. Indeed, a 1993 national inquiry into the human rights of the mentally ill found that older people with mental illness were likely to be ignored by the health care system (Human Rights and Equal Opportunity Commission, 1993). If aged care has often been considered an unfashionable area of nursing practice, this has particularly been so for older people with mental health problems. While this situation is lamentable in respect of the professional priorities of individual nurses, demographic trends—an ageing population and rising acuity levels—indicate that such neglect may well prove disastrous in the first few decades of the new century (Edwards, 1996).

In this chapter, it is assumed that the majority of nurses working in Australia are likely, at some stage in their career, to be called upon to provide nursing care for older people experiencing some form of mental disorder. The capacity to carry out a comprehensive assessment of the mental health of an older person should thus be considered an essential part of the performance capability of all nurses, and not just those working in specialised mental health or aged care services. Accordingly, this chapter outlines the components of a comprehensive mental health assessment for an older person. While specialised assessment instruments are often used in mental health or aged care services (eg, Clifton Assessment Procedures for the Elderly (CAPE), in Pattie and Gilleard, 1979) this chapter focuses instead on the knowledge and skills required to recognise (and thus respond to) mental health problems and disorders experienced by older people in any health care setting.

The next section introduces the theoretical and conceptual bases to mental health assessment, and provides a brief overview of the most common mental disorders found in older people. It has long been known that health (and other) professionals can label people in ways that have serious social implications, and that this is a particular issue for mental health services. Older people may face the double jeopardy of discrimination arising from both ageism and the stigma associated with mental illness. Labels such as 'old' and 'mentally ill' can have serious consequences for how a person is perceived by their family and friends, by health professionals and in the wider community. These issues are briefly addressed in the second section of the chapter. The third section outlines what should be covered in a comprehensive mental health assessment of an older person, including baseline demographic data, functional status, satisfaction with life, mental status and psychiatric symptoms. The chapter concludes with a brief discussion of the relationship between mental health assessment and the evaluation of mental health outcomes, approaching this from the perspective of evidence-based practice.

mental disorder in the older person

Reed and Clarke (1999) have recently noted that while older people with health problems are often talked *about* by health professionals, they are rarely talked *to*. Indeed, family members are frequently preferred as a source of information on the health problems of the elderly, rather than consulting the elderly person themselves. Dismissing the voice of older people too easily can result in inappropriate and ineffective care (ibid., p. 173). A non-inclusive approach to assessing a person's health needs can result in a failure to appreciate an individual's personal experience of illness. It is important to balance practicality, warmth, sensitivity and thoroughness in assessing the mental health of a person who is in a very vulnerable and disorganised state (Weir and Oei, 1996, p. 167).

While older people can be affected by any of the major forms of mental disorder, much of the recent literature on the mental health of older citizens tends to concentrate on two main areas: dementia and depression. In identifying elderly people as a group with particular vulnerabilities, the Human Rights and Equal Opportunity Commission (1993, p. 509) singled out depression and dementia as two disorders that 'afflict [the elderly] particularly frequently'.

depression

A depressed mood and a loss of interest or pleasure are the major symptoms of depression. People experiencing depression report feeling hopeless, worthless, 'blue' or 'down in the dumps'. Other features of the condition include insomnia, weight loss or weight gain, significantly reduced physical activity (often known as psychomotor retardation), diminished ability to think and concentrate, and recurrent thoughts of death. Around two-thirds of depressed patients contemplate suicide, with about 10 to 15 per cent committing it (Kaplan and Sadock, 1991, pp. 366–7). The incidence of depression in the elderly is difficult to calculate as the condition is often diagnosed incorrectly (Edwards, 1996, p. 284). Nevertheless, even conservative estimates suggest that in excess of 100 000 elderly Australians may be affected. Moreover, depression often accompanies other health problems, including dementia. To complicate matters further, depressive symptoms are not uncommon as medication side effects in the elderly. While depression is often associated with positive treatment outcomes in mental health care, the condition is often overlooked in the elderly (Human Rights and Equal Opportunity Commission, 1993, p. 511).

dementia

While 'dementia' is commonly taken to refer to the progressive and irreversible loss or impairment of mental powers, health professionals associate the term with a group of conditions in which the most prominent symptoms are memory loss and confusion, sometimes accompanied by delusions, gross changes in personality and depression.

Approximately 70 per cent of cases of dementia are due to Alzheimer's disease; however, dementia can also result from conditions such as AIDS, Parkinson's disease, stroke, and alcohol-induced and other forms of brain damage. While it is the most common mental health problem in those aged 80 and above, dementia is also a significant problem in those aged 65 to 80. Population projections for Australia (and comparable nations) suggest the likelihood of a marked increase in the numbers of dementia sufferers in the coming decades (up to 16 per cent of the population will be affected by 2021). In most industrialised nations, dementia currently affects around 5 per cent of those aged over 65. However, the incidence rises sharply as age increases; by age 80 and above, 20 per cent are affected. It is expected that within a decade as many as 200000 people in Australia will suffer from dementia (up from around 100000 to 140000 in the mid-1990s) (Human Rights and Equal Opportunity Commission, 1993, pp. 509–10).

interview technique in mental health assessment

Assessment in mental health provides information to determine needs and problems requiring attention, to formulate nursing care, and to evaluate the outcomes of treatment. In this regard, it utilises the steps of the problem-solving model illustrated in Chapter 1. The assessment of a person's mental health incorporates several different forms of data gathered from different sources. Nurses working with elderly (and other) clients in mental health settings can employ a variety of basic methods of assessment, including structured and unstructured interviews, direct observation and the use of standardised assessment instruments. Nowadays, most assessment protocols are standardised to some extent and comprise both structured and unstructured components.

Standardised assessment protocols generally consist of a series of questions to be covered. While these allow consistency in data collection techniques, questions are nevertheless restricted to those listed in the guide, a shortcoming when the person being interviewed presents with data not covered in the interview protocol. For this reason, it is a good idea to include additional unstructured interview techniques (Rapp and Wilcox, 1985). It has been suggested that questions focusing on behaviour are often a good starting point as these are generally easy to answer. Similarly, the most difficulty is likely to be encountered in respect of questions regarding feeling states because of the highly complex and subjective nature of these. The careful ordering of questions can assist in making the person being interviewed feel comfortable (ibid., p. 70).

The phrasing of questions is also an important consideration. Getting the person to describe what has caused them to present is a useful strategy (eg, Describe what has been happening to you. When did these problems begin? Has anything like this happened before? What do you do when you become depressed?). The person being interviewed can also be asked to quantify their answers (eg, rate your discomfort on a scale of one to ten when you feel anxious). Interviewers can also begin to gain an appreciation of the person's perception of the problem by asking what they think the problem is, and what would have to happen for the problem to be improved or controlled. However, asking the questions is only the beginning; attending carefully to what is said and how it is said are equally important. Tone of voice, rate of speech and voice volume can all indicate psychopathology. Similarly, careful observation of the person's posture, gestures, behaviour and appearance during the interview can produce important data (Rapp and Wilcox, 1985).

what should be assessed?

The bio-psycho-social model provides the conceptual starting point for a comprehensive approach to assessing and treating mental health problems and disorders. As Weir and Oei (1996, p. 162) indicate, this covers three broad integrating dimensions of a person's functioning:

- biological functioning (physical or organic processes)
- psychological functioning (mental functioning, including thought, emotion, and behaviour) and
- social functioning (sociability, including interactions with family, friends, work and professional colleagues).

The various health problems that nurses may face in working with elderly (and other) people who are mentally ill include limitations of self-care and impaired functioning, emotional stress, changes in self-concept and life process, alterations in cognitive abilities, physical symptoms accompanying altered psychological functioning, and behavioural risks to self and/or others (Weir and Oei, 1996, pp. 165–6).

. The following broad areas (at least) should be considered in conducting a comprehensive mental health assessment on an elderly person:

- Physical functioning: consideration of how effectively the person being assessed performs a range of physical self-care activities provides an approximate measure of the level of independent functioning.
- Psychological functioning: while confusion is perhaps most often thought of when questions of psychological functioning are raised in respect of elderly people, this can result from deficits across a range of psychological functions such as memory, orientation, attention, judgment, intellect and perception.
- Social functioning: the ability to maintain social relationships and emotional ties, and to undertake a range of social functions are

important indicators of a person's ability to maintain home life, social life, political functioning, and to assert themself in pursuing personal goals and objectives, personal care and the other tasks required of an autonomous individual. Among other things, deterioration in social functioning may indicate reduced cognitive and/or physical functioning.

Given the range of physical, psychological and social functions that can be affected by mental health problems, a systematic and comprehensive approach to mental health assessment is required. However, the pressures of routine clinical work also require that the practicality—ease and brevity of use—of an assessment approach be considered. The aims of a comprehensive mental health assessment are to establish the basis for ongoing rapport between the client and the clinician, to gain knowledge of the client's characteristic patterns of living and functioning, to elicit the past history of the client, and to provide an assessment of their cognitive functioning. While there is no single way of undertaking the interview process, most experienced clinicians, and most textbooks covering the topic, point to very similar approaches. Figure 6.1 sets out a possible approach to comprehensive mental health assessment.

The mental status examination (MSE) is an especially important component of any comprehensive mental health assessment. The MSE provides a generally agreed method of organising clinical observations, providing a clinical baseline for the client's psychological state and providing specific information to assist in establishing the nature of a person's mental health problems. Ordinarily undertaken as part of the broader semi-structured mental health assessment interview, the MSE provides a description of a person's present appearance, demeanour, speech, actions and thoughts.

While variations in format occur from one experienced practitioner to another, all versions of the MSE nevertheless seek certain categories of information. Table 6.1 sets out a typical format for the MSE, based on an approach described by Kaplan and Sadock (1991, pp. 201–4); it is organised under the dimensions of general description, mood and affect, speech, perceptual disturbances, thought, sensorium and cognition, impulse control, judgment and insight, and reliability.

Time constraints and practicality requirements in routine clinical practice have led to the development of abbreviated versions of the MSE, the mini mental state examination (MMSE). In broad terms, a MMSE can

Demographic data:
Name, sex, age, date of birth, marital status, living situation, and religion of family members.
Intake data:
Date and time of presentation, admission, or intake; type of admission; order under the Mental Health Act (if appropriate).
Reason for intake:
Current problems as perceived by consumer.
Previous mental health history:
Dates, inpatient/outpatient treatment, reasons for and types of treatment, effectiveness of treatments.
Drug and/or alcohol use:
Amount, frequency, duration of past and present use of legal and illegal substances, date and time of last use.
Disturbances in daily life functioning:
Sleep, diet, elimination, sexual activity, work, leisure, self-care, hygiene, autonomous functioning.
Social support:
Amount of social contact, nature and quality of relationships, availability of support.
MSE/MMSE
General appearance: type and condition of clothing, cleanliness, physical condition, posture.
Behaviours *during interview:* anger, cooperativeness, evasiveness, withdrawal, motor activity (restlessness, agitation, lack of activity), speech patterns.
Orientation: time, place, person, level of consciousness.
Memory: recent and remote, blackouts, confabulation.
Thought processes reflected in speech: blocking, circumstantiality, loose associations, tangential ideas, ambivalence.
Thought content: helplessness, hopelessness, worthlessness, guilt, suicidal ideas or plans, suspiciousness, phobias, obsessions, preoccupations, antisocial ideas.
Hallucinations: visual, auditory.
Delusions: of reference, influence, persecution, grandeur, religious.
Intellectual functioning: use of language and knowledge, abstract versus concrete thinking (proverbs), calculation (serial sevens).
Affect/mood: anxiety level, elevated or depressed mood, blunted or flat affect, inappropriate affect.
Insight: degree of awareness of problems and their causes.
Judgment: soundness of problem solving and decision making.
Motivation: degree of motivation for treatment.

Figure 6.1: *An approach to comprehensive mental health assessment*

be thought of as measuring cognitive impairment. Besides taking no more than ten to fifteen minutes to administer, the MMSE is relatively easy to use. While a number of variants exist, most are similar to that developed by Jorm (1987, cited in Arthur, Dowling and Sharkey, 1992, p. 148) (see Figure 6.2). This version comprises a series of straightforward questions in the dimensions of orientation, registration, attention and calculation, recall and language, for which answers are scored as correct or incorrect.

Table 6.1: *Typical format for the MSE*

General description	General characteristics—appearance, conduct, attitude—that appear outstanding to the interviewer (eg, posture, poise, clothing, grooming, mannerisms, gestures, twitches, agitation, cooperativeness, friendly, frank, seductive, hostile, evasive).
Mood, affect and appropriateness	Subjective and objective manifestations of the person's emotional state. Mood refers to the pervasive and sustained emotion influencing the person's perception of the world. Affect refers to the external expression of emotional responsiveness. Appropriateness refers to the congruence of emotional response to context (eg, depressed, irritable, euphoric, perplexed, frightened, guilty, constricted, flattened, blunted).
Speech	Physical characteristics—rate, quantity and quality—of speech (eg, talkative, taciturn, rapid, slow, mumbled, loud).
Perceptual disturbances	Presence of hallucinations and/or illusions. Hallucinations are false perceptions in any of the senses. Illusions are mistaken perceptions (eg, hearing voices, experiencing false tastes and smells).
Thought	Disturbances in the way in which ideas and associations are put together (ie, in the process or form of thought). Disturbances in what the person is thinking about (ie, in the content of thought), such as over-abundance or poverty of ideas, rapid thinking, slow or hesitant thinking, ideas which are poorly associated, delusions, preoccupations, obsessions, compulsions, phobias.
Sensorium and cognition	The person's state of consciousness and ability to perceive the environment accurately: *Level of consciousness*, or awareness of the environment (eg, fluctuating awareness of environment). *Orientation*, or awareness of time, place, and person (eg, impaired sense of time, place or person). *Memory*, including remote memory, recent past memory, recent memory and immediate retention and recall (eg, impaired recent memory and immediate retention and recall). *Concentration*, or ability to concentrate on a cognitive task (eg, accurately subtracting seven backwards from 100 repeatedly accurately (serial seven test)). *Abstract thinking*, or ability to deal effectively with concepts and ideas (eg, explaining simple proverbs such as

Table 6.1: *Continued*

	'people who live in glass houses shouldn't throw stones'). *Fund of information and intelligence,* or capacity for simple problem solving, (eg, impaired basic mental tasks such as counting correct change from a simple money transaction), general knowledge appropriate to educational and cultural background (eg, naming recent prime ministers).
Impulse control	Ability to control sexual, aggressive and other impulses (eg, awareness of socially appropriate behaviour and estimation of potential danger to self and others).
Judgment and insight	Capability for *social judgment,* or ability to understand the likely outcome of certain types of behaviour (eg, how a person might act in an imaginary situation such as smelling smoke in a movie theatre). Level of *insight,* or the understanding a person has of their problem; how it affects their feelings, thoughts, behaviours, and judgment.
Reliability	The interviewer's assessment of the person's reliability and capacity to report his or her situation accurately.

(Adapted from Kaplan and Sadock, 1991, pp. 201–204)

mental health assessment and evaluation of outcomes

Among other things, assessment can provide useful data upon which to base judgments regarding how well a person is responding to treatment. As with other areas of health care, those working in mental health are responding to calls for a more systematic approach to evaluating the outcomes (for consumers) of mental health care. One requirement for making a judgment regarding the attribution of an outcome to an intervention or a service is the availability of valid and reliable data regarding the person's condition prior to, during and following the implementation of a treatment regimen (Andrews, Peters and Teesson, 1994). The widespread adoption in routine clinical practice of standardised instruments such as the MSE and the MMSE will certainly assist in the move towards evidence-based practice (Farrell, 1997; Hazelton and Farrell, 1998).

Orientation (10 points)
What is the year?
What is the season?
What is the day of the week?
What is the month?
Can you tell me where we are? (residence or street name required)
What city or town are we in?
What state are we in?
What country are we in?
What are the names of two streets nearby?
What floor of the building are we on?
Registration (3 points)
I am going to name three objects. After I have said them, I want you to repeat them. Remember what they are because I am going to ask you to repeat them in a few minutes. 'Apple . . . Table . . . Penny'.
Attention and calculation (5 points)
Can you subtract seven from 100, and subtract seven from the answer you get and then subtract seven until I tell you to stop?
Now I am going to spell a word forwards and I want you to spell it backwards (in reverse order). W . . . O . . . R . . . L . . . D (D . . . L . . . R . . . O . . . W).
(score the highest of either of these)
Recall (3 points)
What were the three objects I asked you to remember?
Language (9 points)
What is this called? (show watch)
What is this called? (show pencil)
Please repeat the following phrase after me: 'No ifs and buts'.
Read the words on this page and then do what it says ('Close your eyes').
Take this paper in your right hand, fold the paper in half using both hands, and put the paper down using your left hand (3 points).
Pick up the paper and write a short sentence (sentence must have a subject and a verb and make sense).
Now copy the design you see on the page (the design is interlocking pentagons. The result must have five-sided figures with intersection forming a four-sided figure).
Scoring
24–30: no cognitive impairment
18–23: mild cognitive impairment
17 or less: severe cognitive impairment
(Jorm, 1987, cited in Arthur, Dowling & Sharkey, 1992: 148)

Figure 6.2: *Typical format for the MMSE*

conclusion

Depression and dementia are common mental health disorders that affect elderly people. This is of particular concern since many mental health professionals display therapeutic pessimism in relation to elderly people with mental illness.

Comprehensive mental health assessment is used to establish the basis for ongoing rapport between the client and the clinician, to gain knowledge of characteristic patterns of living and functioning as a citizen, and to elicit the past history of the client and provide an assessment of their cognitive functioning. The primary assessment tool is the mental status examination (MSE). All versions of the MSE include the areas of general description, mood, affect, speech, perceptual disturbances, thought, sensorium, cognition, impulse control, judgment, insight and reliability. Time constraints and practicality requirements in routine clinical practice have led to the development of brief versions of the MSE, known as mini mental state examinations (MMSEs).

study questions

1   With reference to Dora's case study below, and using the approach to comprehensive mental health assessment that is set out in Table 1, answer the following questions:

   a   What do you know about the level of social support available to Dora?

   b   Identify the range of disturbances to Dora's daily functioning.

   c   Using the MSE format set out in Table 6.1, identify the extent of disturbance to Dora's mental state.

   d   To what extent should you be concerned at the score of nine obtained using the MMSE? Why?

   e   What other forms of information might you need to develop a comprehensive understanding of Dora's mental health problems?

2   Given Dora's condition, you may find it difficult to administer some sections of the MMSE as set out in Figure 6.2. How would you deal with this, while still conducting a mental status examination?

3   What do you think is the most likely explanation for Dora's condition?

4   What other possible explanations might be supported by the assessment data you have generated?

5.   How would you go about explaining the findings of your assessment to Dora's son and daughter-in-law?

case study: Dora

Dora is 87 years of age. She was born in rural New South Wales and spent most of her life living and working on various cattle stations with her husband Mack. Mack died 18 years ago of a heart attack. Following Mack's death, and with the assistance of several of her children, Dora moved into town, to a single bedroom self-contained unit situated within a retirement village. She lived there happily for many years; two of her five children also live in the district and they visited her regularly.

Her oldest living son and his wife live in Sydney and Dora has visited them for several weeks on an annual basis for many years.

Apart from arthritis (which has worsened significantly in recent years), Dora has enjoyed good health all her life. She has never smoked, very rarely drinks alcohol and has no history of mental illness. Several months ago, Dora had a hip replacement on the left side. While the operation seemed to go well, Dora was very slow to recover and never regained the level of mobility expected. It became clear that she would not be able to care for herself when discharged from hospital. Following family consultations, it was decided that she would go to live with her son in Sydney.

Dora was moved to Sydney almost three months ago and now lives with her son and daughter-in-law (who both recently retired). She is visited by a community nurse on a daily basis, but has mainly been cared for by her daughter-in-law. While Dora's health problems initially seemed to be physical in nature, other problems have since developed. While she can recognise and remembers the names of close family members such as her children and their partners, Dora increasingly has difficulty remembering the names of her grandchildren and great-grand-children. She is often unsure of the time of day and day of the week. On a number of occasions (especially at night) she has seemed to think she was back in her retirement unit. On several occasions, Dora has called out to Mack to come and help her.

Dora can now use a walking frame, but cannot find the toilet, despite having been familiar with the internal layout of her son's home for many years. Dressing and basic hygiene also cause difficulties; if her clothes are not set out Dora is unable to manage simple tasks such as turning the sleeves of a blouse the correct way out. While her speech makes sense, Dora speaks very softly and slowly and sometimes repeats the same things over again. She frequently falls asleep in the middle of the day, but also sleeps through most of the night. She cries frequently at different times of the day and night and has been incontinent of urine and faeces more often in the last month than was the case previously. She was recently assessed as having an MMSE score of nine.

references

Andrews, G., Peters, L. and Teesson, M. (1994), 'The measurement of consumer outcome in mental health: A report to the National Mental Health Information Strategy Committee', Clinical Research Unit for Anxiety Disorders, Sydney.

Arthur, D., Dowling, J. and Sharkey, R. (1992), *Mental Health Nursing. Strategies for Dealing with the Difficult Client*, W. B. Saunders/Bailliere Tindall, Sydney.

Australian Health Ministers (1998), *Second National Mental Health Plan*, Mental Health Branch, Commonwealth Department of Health and Family Services, Canberra.

Edwards, H. (1996), 'Older people' in M. Clinton and S. Nelson (eds), *Mental Health and Nursing Practice*, Blackwell Science, Sydney, pp. 275–92.

Farrell, G. (1997), *Getting up to Speed with Evidence-Based Practice*, Australian and New Zealand College of Mental Health Nurses, Greenacres, South Australia.

Hazelton, M. and Farrell, G. (1998), *Evaluating the Outcomes of Mental Health Care: An Introduction*, Australian and New Zealand College of Mental Health Nurses, Greenacres, South Australia.

Human Rights and Equal Opportunity Commission (1993), *Human Rights and Mental Illness. Report of the Inquiry into the Human Rights of People with Mental Illness* (two volumes), Australian Government Publishing Service, Canberra.

Kaplan, H. I. and Sadock, B. J. (1991), *Synopsis of Psychiatry. Behavioural Sciences. Clinical Psychiatry*, 6th edn, Williams and Wilkins, Baltimore.

Pattie, A. H. and Gilleard, C. J. (1979), *Manual of the Clifton Assessment Procedures for the Elderly (CAPE)*, Hodder and Stoughton Educational, Sevenoaks, UK.

Rapp, S. and Wilcox, S. (1985), 'Methods of assessment in psychiatric nursing' in B. Backer, P. Dubbert and E. E. Senman (eds), *Psychiatric/Mental Health Nursing*, Wadsworth Health Division, California, pp. 68–75.

Reed, J. and Clarke, C. (1999), 'Older people with mental health problems: Maintaining a dialogue' in M. Clinton and S. Nelson (eds), *Advanced Practice in Mental Health Nursing*, Blackwell Science, Sydney, pp. 173–93.

Weir, D. and Oei, T. (1996), 'Mental disorder: Conceptual framework, classification and assessment' in M. Clinton and S. Nelson (eds), *Mental Health and Nursing Practice*, Blackwell Science, Sydney, pp. 161–79.

chapter 7

assessing environment

Bridget Sutherland

chapter summary

This chapter examines the concept of environment and offers a way of understanding some of the complexities involved in assessment of this area of an older person's life. Examples are offered to assist in systemically approaching comprehensive assessments of the lifestyle patterns that are influenced by the environment.

objectives

After reading and reflecting on this chapter, you will be able to:

- identify the factors constituting 'environment'
- analyse the relationship between a person and their environment
- examine the factors involved in assessment of the environment.

introduction

defining the environment

In the context of this chapter, the word 'environment' refers to an older person's habitat, whether the person is residing in their own home or in an aged care facility. The environment or habitat therefore encompasses a person's surroundings—the interior and the exterior of their place of residence and its place in the local neighbourhood.

sense of place

Above all, the place of residence is a 'home', variously described as 'where the heart is', 'the heart of life' and 'be it ever so humble, there's no place like home'. This is where a person feels at ease, belongs and, if possible, is able to create surroundings that reflect their own taste and pleasure and convey a sense of place.

A home has to accommodate a broad range of activities, from sleeping and cooking to relaxing with friends and family. It is a repository for all kinds of equipment, provisions and possessions. In older age, needs alter and there are changes of use and emphasis that require careful planning, efficient servicing and sensible, flexible organisation.

ageing in place—independently

One of the aims of caring for independent older people is to develop respect for their individuality and independence while helping them face the difficulties encountered in their environment. Most OECD (Organisation for Economic Cooperation and Development) countries have been pursuing policies that present people with choice in making decisions about their living arrangements. Many of these policies have the intended effect of maintaining as many people as possible in their own homes. Victoria's 'Ageing in Place' is an example of such a policy. The Victorian Department of Human Services believes Ageing in Place incorporates a mix of service responses under a coherent policy framework. The major areas of policy are housing, urban design, transport, home-care, delivery of health services (eg, 'ambulatory care centres', Hospital in the Home, the Post-Acute Care Program) and public safety (policing, road safety, crime prevention). However, Ageing in Place principles must incorporate the availability of and access to a range of services, including mainstream health services as well as specialised long-term care services.

The increasing focus on ageing in place, whether a person's condition is characterised by wellness, frailty or disability, is making diverse demands on the capacity of the environment to be adapted to meet specific needs. Homes are now being modified, not only to assist the primary occupant directly, but also to facilitate other users such as paid and/or voluntary carers and health care professionals delivering treatment in the home.

the nurse and assessment of the home environment

The terms 'health professional', 'health care visitor' and 'carer', for the purpose of this chapter, are synonymous with the term 'nurse'. Nurses may be members of different teams, such as those provided by:

- the Commonwealth Aged Care Assessment Service (or ACAT: aged care assessment team), supported by the Department of Human Services
- community health services or centres (state Aged and Disability Services)
- local council home-care services
- the Royal District Nursing Service
- other private agencies (eg, privately operated home nursing services).

The general training nurses undertake should provide them with the necessary skills to conduct a general assessment of the level of care needs, including safety risk factors, associated with an older person's living environment. This applies whether the nurse is a member of a multi-disciplinary team (comprising, for example, occupational therapist, community nurse, physiotherapist, podiatrist and social worker) or is acting independently.

For the health care professional, a visit to an older person in their own home, whether for assessment or treatment, demands the observance of certain protocols that can best be described as 'good manners' (see Chapter 5 'Social and lifestyle assessment' for more discussion on this topic). The health care visitor is, after all, entering someone's special place and questions such as, 'Where should I put my coat?' (there being no visible suitable spot), 'Is it all right to put my case on this table?' (the table may have just been cleaned and the case may not be clean) and 'Is it convenient to enter the bedroom now?' (the bedroom is a very private space) are examples of appropriate social behaviour under these circumstances.

Before assessing the necessary physical adaptations or modifications to the home, the older person's mobility and cognitive awareness need to be evaluated. With older age, people often become more set in their ways, so observation of their customary habits is very important, such as:

- How does the older person use the items within their house (eg, are the chairs solid and firm enough to lean on without tipping over?).
- Where do they keep their medication and items like glasses and keys?
- Is the level of lighting adequate—inside and outside?
- Have they had any falls, and, if so, do they remember where and how?
- Are they wearing an 'Alert' button and does it work?

Even though the home may have been previously assessed for safety issues, the health care professional must also recognise and handle potential environmental hazards on each visit. Internally, grease may have been spilt on the kitchen floor, electric cords may be dangling dangerously across a sink, or the resident's favourite loose mat with a toe-catching curled edge may have been replaced after the occupational therapist had ensured it was stowed away on the last visit. The loose mat perceived as a hazard may be, in fact, a valued family possession. There may also be a valid reason for its being there, as it is acting as a marker, particularly if the older person is visually impaired. Visually impaired people need to have markers around the house.

Externally, the garden approach pathway may be slippery because of moss and damp leaves and the globe for the outside sensor light may need replacing. Cracked and broken paths are also hazardous, as are non-aligned pavers or bricks. Assessment of the home environment and subsequent changes require great sensitivity on the part of the health care visitor. Items deemed to be dangerously cluttering up the home may well be the loved collectables of a lifetime. Any changes, such as altering the position of furniture, should be introduced with great caution otherwise there is the potential for confusion on the part of the resident.

continuing assessment of the home environment

Continuing assessment of the home environment from the nursing perspective involves the eight-step problem solving model illustrated in Chapter 1, through the following:

- Reporting to team managers and service providers.
- Updating case documentation: do the nurse and other carers have access to the original report?
- Continuing observation of the home environment, possibly revealing new hazards unnoticed at the time of the original assessment.
- Case conferences: does the team meet on a regular basis to discuss the older person's needs—'What is happening now?', 'What should happen?'.
- Has the care plan been discussed with the older person and other people (eg, family members) in residence.
- Dealing with problems such as an older person suffering from cardiovascular problems due to physical frailty, who is living alone in a block of flats without a lift and who is unable to cope with walking up and down flights of stairs. Under such circumstances, a visit from the ACAS (Commonwealth Aged Care Assessment Service) may be necessary for referral to either respite care or for permanent placement in an aged care facility.

The challenge facing the assessment team in maintaining older people in their own homes, where this is their choice, even in cases where needs are complex and levels of incapacity severe, is to match the physical needs of the older person with their functional needs. Ideally, this is achieved by working with other team members to identify opportunities for continued independence via adapted functional techniques, assistive equipment or home modification.

guidelines for assessing the function and safety of the home environment

entrances

- Security: is there a sensor light? If there is a flywire door, does it close securely? Does the doorbell work? Do keys, bolts or locks for gates, garage and entrances work?
- Are external surfaces slippery? If there are steps, how many are there and are they slippery? Is there a handrail to assist going up and down?

lounge and dining room

- Are the chairs solid and firm enough to lean on without tipping over?
- Are chairs and sofas high enough for comfortable sitting down and getting up?
- Are table lamps sturdy and well balanced?
- Do standard lamps have solid bases to prevent tipping over?
- Is the telephone within easy reach, preferably on a side table beside a chair?
- Are the cords for the telephone and electrical appliances out of harm's way?
- Are there loose mats or rugs to cause slipping and tripping?
- Is the lounge/dining room far from the kitchen?

bedroom

- Is the bed sturdy with an edge firm enough for sitting on? A bed on legs is safer than one on castors (unless castors are lockable).
- Is there access to the sides of the bed and around the bed?
- What is the distance to the bathroom? Is there a need for a commode?
- Is there good lighting in the room and a light beside the bed?
- Is there a telephone beside the bed?
- Are the cords for telephone, lamp, electric blanket and clock radio secure?
- If there is a bedside rug or mat, is it well secured?

bathroom

- Have grab rails been installed? Towel rails are not safe as grab rails.
- Is the floor non-slip?
- Has the base of the bath/shower been rendered non-slip?
- If there is a bath mat, is it non-slip?
- If the resident uses a bath, perhaps a bath board could be installed for easier access.
- Is there thermostatic heating control?
- Is there a safe seat for drying?
- Does the door swing out? If not, perhaps it could be re-hung.

toilet

- Is the seat height adequate, or is a raised toilet seat required?
- Does the door swing out?

kitchen

- Is the lighting adequate?
- Is the height of benches adequate? Is there good access to cupboards, drawers, cooker and pantry?
- Can the appliances be easily operated?
- Are electrical cords secure?
- Is the kitchen reasonably clean, with no dangerous floor spillage?

laundry

- Is the outside access secure?
- Is the path from laundry to clothes line safe?
- Does the resident have a laundry trolley? An adjustable ironing board? A dryer? A clothes horse? Are they are all in a safe condition?
- Are there steps leading down from the laundry door? A ramp is much safer.

ageing in place—residential care

The National Aged Care Strategy, which came into operation on 1 October 1997, combined Australia's traditional system of residential care—nursing homes (for higher dependency residents) and hostels (for lower dependency residents)—into one uniform system. Government policy also focuses on the quality of life for the residents in aged care facilities and the standards against which facilities are assessed and accredited now takes this into account, as well as the integral health care provided.

As far as the actual accommodation is concerned, the emphasis is on creation of a home-like atmosphere with respect to design, furnishings and practices. The design should also assist residents with disabilities and the staff in their care of the residents. Adequate personal space must be available to residents, so that a reasonable number of their own belongings can remain in their possession. The means of protecting these belongings from other residents, who may be intrusive, should also be available.

The challenge for all those involved in facility design is to achieve a balance between an easily cleaned, maintained and safe environment and an environment that is homelike in character. Most of the institutions of the past, where everything from the physical environment to the provision of care appeared totally clinical (or in some older style accommodation, Dickensian), are gone. Those that may still exist will certainly not obtain accreditation under the new Commonwealth program. The following description of an old nursing home bedroom by Ellen Newton (1979, p. 14) illustrates the de-personalised world of the past:

> ... Almost covering the wall at the foot of the bed was a double wardrobe, twice too big for the room. It had been heavily mistreated with a heavy black stain and looked within a couple of feet of the ceiling. The floor was covered with a sallow, mottled linoleum that shone as if it had been lacquered ... and beside the bed, a table that might once have supported an aspidistra. It barely held a spindly metal lamp, a plastic water bottle and a glass ... In the corner nearest my bed was a shabby, dark brown armchair, the size and shape they used to have in the smoke rooms of old country pubs. It looked as if it had been heavily sat on by several generations of broad buttocks ...

the nurse and the residential environment

The decision to enter a facility is very hard for most older people. As well as acceptance of the fact that they can no longer manage, or be managed, to live independently comes the realisation that their mortality is now visible to themselves, their families and neighbours. They must now live in care, probably for the rest of their lives. Once the decision is made, there is the tremendous upheaval of leaving their home, family and friends, let alone their pets.

The following extract from Ronald Blythe (1979, p. 136) provides a vivid description of such a final departure. The narrator is the matron of a county council older people's home in the United Kingdom:

> ... it isn't easy for the person who will eventually make a go of it in the old people's home to give up all they possess. Pack their clothes ... stop the milk, give the cat away, change the address on the pension-book, shut the front door—Oh, just imagine that day ...

Although they are now entering a place that is, to all intents and purposes, regarded as their future 'home', the initial impact of unfamiliar communal living with a perceived loss of privacy must be immense. Isolated from family, friends and pets, and with their personal possessions contained in a bedroom, it is no wonder some older people suffer a loss of personal identity. One resident, who had entered an aged care facility with her husband, confided in me:

> We have been able to bring a few things with us, dear—most importantly for me, some of our pictures. My children have

disposed of everything else; I suppose they kept some pieces of furniture for themselves, but I really don't want to know where they have gone, or who has taken what; it's too sad.

However, not all new residents are so despondent. Mr M was delighted. He was about to enter the recently opened hostel (lower dependency) of an aged care facility where his wife was already living in the established nursing home (higher dependency). After visiting his wife in the nursing home section, he arrived at the hostel, 'driving' his motorised wheelchair with his wheeled walking frame attached behind. The new manager (an RN) greeted him at the door: 'Welcome to your new home, Mr M. Just park over there, and when you have finished, come and see your room. Take your time, there's no rush.'

She waited inside while Mr M parked his vehicle, unloaded his walking frame, took off his hat and entered his new home. The nature of the manager's greeting provides an excellent example of her good manners and understanding of the need to maintain Mr M's independency level.

As far as the nurse is concerned, the same protocols (or 'good manners') as described earlier, under the heading 'The nurse and assessment of the home environment', also apply to visiting a resident's room in a residential care facility. This is now their private space in their new home. It is respectful to knock on their bedroom door before entering and to call residents Mr, Mrs or Miss until or unless they request that their given name be used. It is also most disrespectful to ignore the resident when two or more carers are in the resident's room for the purposes of, say, bed-making. It is very easy to talk together, discussing the events of the previous evening's entertainment, while the resident is present, whether the resident is cognitively aware or cognitively unaware.

In helping a resident adapt to their new situation, similar observations to those used in the home environment also apply, such as:

- Can they manage to open and close their curtains and/or blinds? This is often very difficult for residents with arthritic hands, so the carer may need to perform this task for the resident.
- Does the favourite chair they have brought from home give them sufficient support for lowering and raising comfortably?
- Is the cord of their own table lamp frayed (if the facility does not provide one) and is it sturdy and well balanced? Does the switch work easily?

- Is their clothing suitable? Long, trailing cords on a dressing gown can lead to tripping, accidents and falls.

Provision of adequate meeting areas for visitors is very important. Quieter sitting areas are usually provided in modern facilities, away from the noise of the television set and the general hurly-burly associated with the everyday operation of the building. The architectural design for a recently completed (August 1998) Hostel at Croydon in Melbourne incorporates a special dining/sitting area for residents, families and friends. Bookings for family functions were made as soon as the first residents moved in.

continuing assessment of the residential care environment

Continuing assessment of the residential care environment involves the same skills and teamwork as for the home environment. Does the care plan include the following, for example:

- How is the resident adapting to their new environment?
- Are they managing to cope with their equipment such as walking frame or wheelchair?
- Are there problems within the environs of the facility that discourage the resident's physical independence and mobility?
- Are maintenance problems such as damaged window furnishings or electrical equipment being attended to promptly?
- What does the resident perceive as their environmental needs?
- Organising feedback from carers, residents and residents' families. What works and what doesn't? Are there any serious complaints?
- Are visitors being encouraged?
- Are the residents being empowered by extending the boundaries of their environment into the local community with visits to the shops, pubs, local parks (particularly those with children's playgrounds) and so on?

Every Wednesday some wheelchair bound residents from a high dependency facility in a Melbourne suburb are taken to lunch at their local pub. Everyone is dressed and groomed for an outing and an air of excitement pervades the facility entrance foyer prior to departure. This excursion is the highlight of these residents' week and provides them with a truly empowering experience.

The priority and challenge for carers are to ensure that respect for the privacy, personhood, dignity and quality of life of people in their care is maintained at all times.

design recommendations from the nursing perspective

Facility design committees necessarily require people with different conceptual skills and experience. Most nurses do not possess the generic skills to design a building. By the same token, most architects do not possess the hands-on experience of working in an aged care facility.

Examples of design deficiencies observed by nurses in modern facilities include:

- Doors that are not wide enough for bed moving. (In one instance, this fault was the result of poor communication between architects and client. The director of nursing presumed the architect was aware of the need for hospital width doors in view of the requirements for respite care and ageing in place. The building was designed for lower level dependency residents and the architect was unaware that wider doors would be needed.)
- Poor or non-existent storage.
- Poorly designed dining rooms with lack of flexibility in meeting residents' dining requirements and no separation of severely disturbed residents from those that are higher functioning.
- Floor coverings that do not suit the level of functioning and incontinence of residents.
- Manager's office situated too close to the entrance and main living area, with resultant lack of privacy for the manager and interviewees. (The position of the office in relation to rest of the building was determined before the appointment of the manager.)
- Internal distances that are too great for the staff to walk.
- Furniture that is ergonomically incorrect. For example:
  - unsuitable seating (too low, too soft and too deep for older people)
  - tables, benches, bed ends and bedside units with sharp corners
  - dining chairs without arms
  - domestic type beds without lockable castors.

The avoidance of the above listed problems, and the many more unlisted, lies in adequate planning at the design stage.

guidelines for the assessment of proposed architectural plans and furnishing fit-out for an aged care facility

interior

Bedrooms

- Size of bedrooms to allow for personal effects and bed making.
- Doors hospital width to allow for bed moving.
- Single rooms mostly required with some doubles also available.
- Signposting (personal identifications if possible).
- Appropriate built-in wardrobes and cupboards.
- Appropriate floor coverings.
- Suitable mirrors.
- Windows not to the floor.
- Curtains preferably to the window sill (for safety reasons such as entangling with wheelchairs).
- Hospital beds to have domestic style bed ends.
- Other beds to be domestic type with edges firm enough to sit on and with lockable castors.
- Bedside units to be immovable for residents, but moveable for cleaning.
- A water-resistant finish for bedside units.
- Lighting (sufficient natural, artificial and night lights).

Bedroom en suites

- Doors wide enough for shower chairs.
- Sufficient space for staff-assisted showers and staff rescue of residents.
- Avoidance of self locking-in.
- Stepless showers.
- Available alarm system.
- Taps: quarter turn; thermostatic mixing valves.
- Non-slip floor covering.
- Accessibility of toilet roll from toilet seat.
- Support grab rails.
- Recessed soap holders.
- Adequate drainage and ventilation.

Dining rooms

- Flexibility of space and tables to enable dining in small or larger groups.
- Able to accommodate disabled residents.
- Adequate lighting.
- Control of noise level.
- A separate area for special needs (eg, dementia specific).
- Toilet facilities adjacent to dining area.
- Floor covering: easy to clean and cope with spillages.

Living areas

- Large enough for group activities (eg, church services, visiting, entertainment, TV watching).
- Adequate lighting.
- Ease of cleaning.
- Comfortable and appropriate seating.
- Small sitting or quiet areas with tea-making facilities for entertaining visitors.

Craft room or activity area

- Adequate storage space.
- Trough or sink for 'wet' activities.
- Suitable floor coverings.

Kitchen area

- Storage.
- Bench space.
- Layout.
- Proximity to dining areas.
- Safety.
- Adequate lighting.
- Accessible for deliveries.
- Adequate power (eg, three-phase electricity).

Laundry

- Large enough.
- Commercial size equipment.
- Storage space.

- Bench space adequate for clothes sorting.
- Adequate system for collecting and returning residents' clothing correctly.
- Accessibility.
- Separate small laundry for residents' own washing.

Storage areas

- Adequate for large equipment such as wheelchairs.
- Adequate for cleaners.
- Staff lockers.
- Medication: if installing a Webster system, are cupboards and shelving the correct size and design?

Corridors

- No dead ends.
- Suitable and sufficient hand rails.
- Adequate lighting.
- Suitable floor covering.
- Width: not too narrow, enabling provision of rest areas if possible.
- Colour contrast between walls and floor.

Entrance

- Size of door sufficient for wheelchair access.
- Security: external sensor lights; no steps.
- Attractive and welcoming.
- Proximity to main living area(s).
- Space for seating, enabling residents to observe comings and goings.
- Office or staff station adjacent.

Office or staff station

- Functional and effective.
- Adequate desk space to incorporate computers, fax and so on.

Staff room

- Comfortable chairs.
- Adequate table(s).

- Tea making facility, microwave and so on.
- Proximity to staff lockers.

Hairdressing

- Provision of adequate professional hairdressing chair(s).

exterior

- Design of gardens: need for pathways that lead to a specific point, say, a garden seat.
- Access for residents to gardening: need for raised beds; or to see gardening being done.
- Inclusion of space for outdoor activities such as a BBQ.
- Adequate fencing: provision of screening and climbing plants.
- Choice of plants: attractive, non-toxic.
- Sufficient shaded areas.
- Safety and maintenance: avoidance of slippery leaves.
- A garden shed.
- A drying area for residents' own washing.

common to all areas

Energy efficient design

- Adequate north facing glass, allowing winter sun.
- Decreased glass on south side.
- Correct depth of eaves for summer protection of windows.
- Adequate insulation.
- Adequate ventilation.

Colour schemes

- Need to be soft with pastels such as pink or green, definitely not red or bright colours.
- Also need for colour contrast between walls and doors.

Floor coverings

- Pattern needs to be simple and not busy, with same pattern covering entire floor area.
- Patterned floor coverings combined with a plain covering can appear as a 'step' for the visually and cognitively impaired.

- A variety of floor coverings probably needed, including carpet tiles and vinyl.

Furniture and furnishings

Consideration needs to be given to:

- design and function, including comfort
- structural soundness and safety
- ease of use and access for users and carers
- stability, mobility, immobility
- user friendliness: edges, corners, tactility
- ease of operation (eg, drawers)
- resistance to wear and tear, including heat, body fluids, spillage
- capacity to withstand occasional abuse
- coordination
- flexibility to allow for rearrangement of rooms to suit individual needs
- use of modern health care fabrics
- use of flame retardant window furnishing fabrics.

general guidelines

The process of decision making for the planning and fit out of a facility is difficult. The challenge for management is to achieve an optimum result both in terms of design and cost effectiveness within an established budget.

We are all concerned with getting value for money. Unless the facility is wealthy enough to replace furniture and furnishings before they wear out, thought must be given to purchasing items, which, although domestic in character, meet life expectancy and cost benefit criteria, not cost criteria alone.

It is not only residents and carers who benefit from an attractive and pleasant environment. The residents' families and their other visitors feel more relaxed and happy seeing them in such surroundings.

case study

The following case history illustrates the kind of problems faced by aged care providers when endeavouring to upgrade their existing facilities to meet current accreditation standards.

project: refurbishment of 120-bed aged care hostel

The hostel was opened in the 1970s and is part of an inner city public hospital aged care network, which encompasses psychogeriatric services, aged care assessment teams, day care, acute care, rehabilitation, nursing homes and hostels.

project aims

- To update and upgrade the hostel to provide a home-like yet practical environment.
- By provision of a small 'residential neighbourhoods' approach, to improve the residents' opportunities for, and enjoyment of, social interaction.
- To improve the interior design to provide a safer environment for the residents, particularly the more cognitively unaware, and their carers.
- To meet the challenge of optimum result for the above aims in terms of design and cost effectiveness within an established budget.

method

- Identify problem areas.
- Establish overall master plan.
- Establish budget.
- List immediate priorities.
- Implementation.

problem areas included

- corridors
- lounge/dining room
- residents' bedrooms
- ground floor administration and entrance area
- residents' kitchens
- staff/carers rest and dining areas
- lack of identity between floors
- most of the furniture
- window furnishings
- lift areas.

master plan included

- Establishment of separate 'neighbourhood' identities for each floor (total three floors) by use of colour-coordinated schemes for walls, floors and furnishings.
- Assessment of all existing furniture, seating and built-ins for suitability in terms of accessibility, comfort and safety.
- Improving corridors: laying carpet tiles in lieu of unsuitable vinyl; wall painting; improved residents' ID of bedroom doors.
- Tidying-up external balconies with provision for more outdoor seating, pots and plants.
- Re-flooring residents' kitchens with non-slip vinyl; repairing cupboards.
- Removal and replacement of built-in bedroom furniture; replacement of window furnishings in bedrooms and en suites; replacement of bedroom flooring.
- Improving intimidating ground floor reception area.
- Reorganisation of administration offices to improve working conditions.
- Redecoration of staff areas; provision for upgraded seating, tables and lockers.

Immediate priority: bedrooms and en suites

- Upgrading and replacement of fixed furniture including beds, tables and storage units with sharp edges.
- Wall-fixed tables with inadequate and unsafe fold-up legs; built-in vanities damaged; door handles missing, etc.
- Replacement of slippery, reflective vinyl flooring with carpet tiles.
- Replacement of window furnishings—very poor condition and not flame retardant.
- Replacement of shower curtains.

Immediate priority: residents' kitchens

- Replacement of slippery, reflective vinyl flooring with non-slip vinyl.
- Repair cupboard doors.

Immediate priority: corridors

- Replacement of slippery, reflective vinyl with carpet tiles.
- Provision of 'rest area' seating.
- Provision of adequate ID for bedroom doors.

Immediate priority: lounge and dining area

- Replacement of window furnishings—all in poor condition and non-flame retardant fabrics.
- Improve lighting.

Immediate priority: ground floor administration and entrance area

- Replacement of dangerous, slippery vinyl flooring.

implementation

For a number of reasons, including severe budgetary restraints, implementation of the above work is taking place over a period of time. Also, with the Ageing in Place policy, refurbishment of the bedrooms can only be carried out when a room becomes vacant due to the death of a resident.

conclusion

Despite the problems, this facility has achieved accreditation. The continuing refurbishment has also improved the morale of the residents, their carers and their families.

study questions

1　How would you define the term environment?
2　Identify factors that influence the assessment of the environment.
3　Describe any differences between assessment of the home environment and the residential care environment.
4　What are the responsibilities of the health care professional in determining the most suitable environment for an older person?
5　Analyse the concept of 'place' in terms of residential care.

acknowledgments

Thanks to Jean Campbell, Bill Deveny, Kaye Gallaugher, Evie Gough, Lyn Hornsby, Debra Reid and Jan Roberts.

references

Blythe, R. (1979), *The View in Winter, Reflections on Old Age*, Allen Lane, London, pp. 130, 136.

Newton, E. (1979), *This Bed my Centre*, McPhee Gribble Publishers, Melbourne, p. 14.

further reading

Archibald, P. (1994), 'Looking back to the future with the elderly', *Architect* (Official Journal of the Victorian Chapter of the RAIA), August.

Australian Institute of Health and Welfare/Office for the Aged in the Commonwealth Department of Health and Family (1997), *Older Australia at a Glance*, Australian Institute of Health and Welfare, Canberra.

Bauby, J-D. (1997), *The Diving Bell and The Butterfly*, (translated by J. Leggatt), Fourth Estate, London.

Conran, T. (1994), *The Essential House Book*, Conran Octopus Limited, London, p. 11.

Dinoglobs Syndicate (1993), *What to Prevent in Future Design of Nursing Homes for the Confused Elderly*, Department of Health and Community Services, Victoria, Melbourne.

Donwood Community Aged Care Services Inc., *The Living at Donwood Document: Information for Day to Day Living*, Donwood Community Aged Care Services Inc., Melbourne.

Edmonston, K. and Thang, V. (1997), *Nursing Homes: An Accommodation or Health Care Issue*, Centre for Biomedical Sciences, University of Canberra, Canberra.

Garner, E. (1995), *Stay on your Feet: Information and Suggestions to Help Prevent Falls*, NSW North Coast Public Health Unit (reprinted 1995 by Aged Care Division, Department of Health and Community Services, Victoria).

Hollis, C. (1998), 'Challenging traditions: Social support for the aged in residential facilities', Paper presented at the World Congress of Gerontology, Adelaide.

Hudson, R. and Richmond, J. (1994), *Unique and Ordinary: Reflections on Living and Dying in a Nursing Home*, Ausmed Publications, Melbourne.

Hudson, R. (1998), 'From individual to community: Personhood in residential aged care', Paper presented at AAG National Conference, Melbourne, October.

Murphy, A. and Kerr, M. (1997), *Partnerships do Make a Difference*, Napier Street Hostel and Royal District Nursing Service Case Management Project, Melbourne.

Royal Melbourne Hospital Multi-Disciplinary Improvement Team and Anne Nicholson Enterprises (1997), *The Care Partnership: Communication and Education Strategies for Healthcare Professionals*, Royal Melbourne Hospital, Melbourne.

Sutherland, B. (1997), Submission: Family and Community Development Committee, Victorian Parliamentary Inquiry into Planning for Positive Ageing (Section 8: Building Environment and Physical Infrastructure).

chapter 8

assessment of patterns of body defence and healing

Sally Garratt

chapter summary

This chapter discusses the processes involved in healing, body defence and the impact of stress in older people. Factors that influence the assessment process and identification of pain in older people are identified. Changes in the body due to ageing and to abnormal deviations are presented to highlight the importance of addressing comprehensive assessment of the parameters of health. Understanding the complexity of what is due to age and what is not underpins the success of accurate assessment.

objectives

After reading and reflecting on this chapter, you will be able to:

- identify differences in body defence patterns in older people
- examine patterns of healing in older people
- explore difficulties in the assessment of pain
- discuss the importance of understanding stress reactions in older people
- analyse abnormal processes of tissue growth in older people.

introduction

As the physical–physiological body ages, the ability to withstand attack from both the internal and external environment decreases. Examination of cellular function reveals that a precarious state of balance exists in older people and that they take longer to return to a balanced state after stress. In fact, one of the major principles of gerontology cited in Carotenuto and Bullock (1981, p. 16) is 'with age, the deviations following stress become greater, and the return to optimal levels are slower'. Successful ageing can be seen as the ability to survive stress, perhaps aided by genetic endowment, learning ability and adopting a lifestyle that is concerned with maintaining balance. Stress has been known to affect the immune status of the person. There are age related changes to the immune system that demonstrate that many of the illnesses related to ageing are the direct result of declining immuno-competence (Chandra, 1992). What has not been determined is whether the number of immune cells decreases or the competence of the cells is less. However, there are known factors that affect the functioning of the immune system. Nutritional deficits are one of the main reasons for defective responses in the immune system. Malnutrition, leading to protein deprivation and iron and trace element (mostly zinc) deficiency affects the cells' ability to maintain resistance to invaders. Vitamin deficiencies will also affect cellular responsiveness (ibid.).

Stressors affecting older people are usually those factors that result from sudden changes in their lifestyle such as relocation, bereavement and loss of relationships. The fact that an older person has been coping with life and its resultant stressors for 80 years or more means that they have also developed a range of coping strategies. However, those personal strengths may not be sufficient when many life changes come in conjunction with failing physical health. Bereavement and relocation stress are often related, as after the death of a spouse the surviving person cannot maintain their lifestyle without help, and often this means professional assistance. Loneliness has been associated with a decrease in immune response and depression has major affects (Lueckenotte, 1996).

The assessment of older people should consider their personal reactions to stress that can be observed and noted as determinants of healing and returning to health. Obtaining a comprehensive profile of the older person's usual reactions to stress, identification of the stressful events in their life and the coping strategies they employed to deal with them is a very important part of any history. While older people maintain the same coping strategies they have always had, they may need assistance to develop some new or different ones when facing major life changes. Understanding the unique impact of stress on the older person is essential before strategies can be discussed with them or their families. Often family members do not understand the impact of stress on their loved one, as the older generation have often been the strong, coping heads of the family for everyone else to lean on in times of crisis. Decision making ability in times of stress alters and the person may appear to be physically ill or depressed, often leading to others confusing these symptoms with symptoms of dementia. Understanding the effects of stress and the implications for the immune system is essential for competent assessment in gerontological care.

Health professionals are concerned with identifying factors that delay healing and observing patterns of physiological, emotional and behavioural responses that indicate disruption in the person. The major areas of assessment this chapter addresses are tissue healing, response to pain and abnormal tissue growth. The problem solving approach outlined in Chapter 1 guides this process.

patterns of tissue healing

The largest organ in the body concerned with healing is the integument, or skin. Skin is also the most obvious tissue to show signs of ageing and the ravages of intrinsic and extrinsic abuse. Intrinsic abuse can arise from multiple factors (eg, ingestion of chemicals or medications, lack of hydration, hormone imbalance, nutritional disturbance, smoking, diseased organs, poor blood supply). Extrinsic abuse results from environmental traumas such as exposure to sun, type of work undertaken, pressure, shearing forces, abrasion, chemical application, microbes, excessive wetting, and diseases of the skin or underlying tissues.

Sustained trauma such as exposure to sun results in changes to the skin that are obvious (ie, redness of sunburn, brown colouration, freckles, melanoma, dryness, cracking, flaking, toughening and callous formation). Sustained alterations in fluid dynamics, nutritional intake and poor blood supply are also readily observable (eg, poor turgor, swelling, temperature changes, white or bluish extremities, dryness, flushing and bruising).

Ageing skin does not react well to hostile microbes and invasion is more likely, as cell penetration is easier. The immune response to bacterial invasion in older people is less effective because both T cell and B cell immunity is decreased. This also is associated with the noted increase in auto-immune disease and cancer. The first response of the body to infection is the development of inflammation. Inflammatory responses in older people are slower and less intense (Ferguson and MacLean, 1997). Wounds caused by friction and pressure are therefore more likely to become infected, and lower extremity ulceration is usually chronically infected. Healing, therefore, is usually delayed due to the intrinsic and extrinsic factors affecting skin and the presence of overlying persistent infection.

Changes to this large organ, or integument, are usually readily observable, and with some knowledge of which changes are due to ageing rather than disease, the assessment process should proceed by direct observation, at the same time noting the potential for possible skin trauma due to identified factors in the internal and external environment. Assessment of skin integrity should start in a systematic fashion from the head to the lower extremities. Observable changes are noted and the size of any lesion, colour, odour, or other characteristics are recorded. Potential for pressure ulcer development can be assessed using a range of current tools (eg, Braden scale, Waterlow scale, Norton scale). The Braden scale scores six categories related to pressure ulcer formation:

- sensory perception
- mobility
- moisture
- nutrition
- activity
- friction and shear.

The scores from each item are totalled. The maximum possible score is 23 and older people are at risk if their total score is 16 or less. Individuals who score 17 or above on the scale would not be expected to require routine turning or any other intensive pressure care prevention regimen. Conversely, as the score declines progressively below 16, increasingly intensive skin ulcer prevention regimens become necessary (Braden and Bergstrom, 1987). A useful tool to guide observation and skin assessment is offered in Table 8.1 (see also Appendix 8.1).

Table 8.1: *Skin assessment*

General observations	Description
Colour	Pink, red, cyanotic, pale, yellow
Texture	Coarse, fine, flaky, scales
Turgor	Lax, responds well, slow to return
Hydration	Full tissue, dry and flat, itchy
Specific characteristics	
Growths	Warts, seborrhoeic keratosis, moles,
Rashes	Eczema, psoriasis, dermatitis, scabies
Discolouration	Freckles, stains, nicotine
Infections	Pustules, fistula, cracks
Broken areas	Open wounds, tears, pressure ulcers require specific assessment
Old scars, indentations	Previous surgery, healing
Systemic alterations	
Altered fluid intake	Below 1500 mL daily
Medication	Synergistic and iatrogenic problems
Constipation	Bowel management program
Nutrition	Insufficient protein, carbohydrate, fat
Infections	Other body systems
Stress	Psychological distress
Environmental factors	
Excessive sun	Leathery, coloured skin
Harsh chemical use	Work usage, laundry detergents, altered pH of skin due to contact
Moisture overload	Excessive wetting, urine, sweat

When there is an obvious break in the integrity of the skin and/or deeper tissues, creating a wound, the assessment becomes more complex. The most common wounds in aged care are pressure ulcers or sores, venous ulcers, arterial ulcers, and surgical sites such as stoma or ostomy openings into stomach or bladder. Care of stoma and ostomy sites is undertaken following explicit instruction from the surgeon who made the wound. The subsequent healing around the site ensures a permanent hole develops.

assessment of skin breakdown and wounds

Any break in the skin or underlying tissues is considered to be a wound and should be assessed for treatment and potential for further problems.

A useful strategy is to follow a management protocol commencing on admission or when the break in skin integrity is noticed (see Figure 8.1).

The most common trauma found in older people is a skin tear from extrinsic damage. Most skin tears are superficial and are often due to knocks against hard objects, scratches or poor lifting techniques. All skin tears must be considered as having the potential for infection and development of further invasive tissue damage.

types of skin tears

There are two main types of skin tears:

- Abrasions (scrapes) are irregular superficial open wounds which are very painful and prone to infection; nerve endings can be exposed.

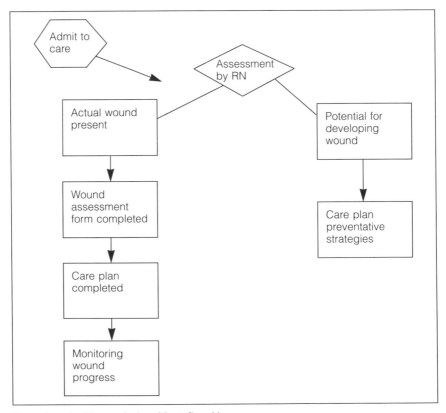

Reproduced with permission, Montefiore Homes

Figure 8.1: *Wound management protocol flow chart*

- Incised tears are cleanly cut and tidy with no bruising or crushing to wound margins. They tend to gape open.

A general assessment of skin tears can be made through the following questions:

- Is there much bleeding?
- Are there foreign bodies in the wound (eg, grease, dirt or gravel)?
- Is the tear dirty? If so, clean with appropriate solutions, then rinse off the cleansing solution with normal saline as cleansing agents have a retarding effect on the healing process.
- Is the tear already showing infection?
- Should consideration be given to prophylactic treatment against tetanus for dirty lesions?
- Are there skin tags that should be removed with sterile scissors?
- Can the tear surfaces be pulled together with wound closure or butterfly strips for incised tears and be covered with clear film dressing? Clear film dressing can be used directly over open tears. A small to moderate amount of exudate is helpful in the healing process. Excessive exudate causes maceration, skin breakdown and infection and should be removed and the dressing changed.

Cellulitis, due to trauma of the damaged skin tissue and infection, can complicate a simple skin tear. Observe for redness, heat, swelling, pain and other signs and symptoms of infection. Treatment is with antibiotics and an appropriate wound dressing.

pressure ulcers

formation of pressure ulcers

Pressure ulcers form easily in older people. Certain factors are believed to predispose a person to pressure ulcer formation. These factors may be either intrinsic (factors that pertain to the person) or extrinsic (factors that pertain to the external environment) (see Figure 8.2).

prediction instrument for pressure ulcers

Each older person in care should be assessed for predisposing susceptibility to pressure ulcers as a routine preventative measure. To assist identification and clinical assessment of residents at risk, scales have been developed to evaluate clinical situations that contribute to the formation of pressure ulcers. The Braden scale (Braden and Bergstrom, 1987) can be used to objectively guide the decision-making process as to

Intrinsic factors	Extrinsic factors
Age Neurological disease Sleep and rest Body type and weight Reduced mobility Skin condition Mental status Nutrition Dehydration Incontinence	External restraints to movement Poor lifting technique or resident handling techniques Inappropriate positioning Poor hygiene Inappropriate clothing Drugs Moisture Pressure Friction Shearing force

Figure 8.2: *Factors that predispose a person to pressure ulcer formation*

which person requires pressure care and which person should be regarded as having the potential for pressure damage. Other scales are available such as the Norton scale and the Waterlow scale.

Once a wound has been identified, the assessment process can be guided by the use of a good reliable assessment tool (see Figure 8.1 and Appendix 8.2). The treatment is decided and ongoing monitoring must be continued until the wound has healed. Monitoring may also be done using the tool illustrated in Appendix 8.2.

patterns of response to pain

There are many myths about the phenomenon of pain and older people. One of these myths centres on the belief that all older people can expect pain from just 'old age' and that a stoic attitude of endurance should exist. The fact that joints wear out and muscles lose power contributes to the notion that old bodies are bound to have more discomfort than younger ones. The older person is more likely to have some form of arthritis; however, that does not condemn them to a life of 'endurance'. Older people feel pain in the same way as any other person feels pain. The neural pathways are the same and the receptor sites translating pain messages do so in the same way as they do in younger people. Responses to pain, however, may differ as pain is very much a phenomenon of the person experiencing it. Older people have a lifetime of experience and most have experienced pain of some intensity for many reasons. Pain may be physical, emotional or spiritual and is a complex experience that draws on past knowledge, physical disruption and culturally expected responses. Acute physical pain is in response to stimulation of nerve pathways by trauma. Infections cause pain by oedema surrounding the receptor sites, chemical stimulation and release of toxins (Groer and Shekelton, 1979).

Acute pain is a protective mechanism for humans, as it occurs when tissue or the psyche is damaged and tells the sufferer to remove the causing stimulus, if possible. How the person reacts is determined by many factors (eg, culture, tolerance levels, physical capability to move, relationships with others, reactions to disease processes and expectations established by health care professionals).

If a carer does not believe the older person has pain when they say they have, a distrust is immediately established that precludes obtaining pain relief. Older people can be more stoic than younger people and can cover up severe pain by ignoring it; they may not wish to seek help from others because they fear a loss of independence, and may not bring their pain to the attention of others because of fear of being rejected.

Older people can mask quite severe pain, and infection or disease can remain undetected until severe health problems are evident. The pain of acute appendicitis is an example. Because the afferent pathways are slower to conduct, the receptor sites have altered, or reactions are tempered by psychological control, appendicitis is often thought to be constipation and misdiagnosed until severe complications arise. Older people who are confused or cognitively impaired may express pain in various ways, usually only detected by those who know them best. Changes in behaviour and responses to stimuli alter because of pain; however, interpreting these changes is difficult and relies on the elimination of other causative factors. For example, if an older man who is demential, but is usually mobile and friendly, and who readily eats his meals, suddenly stops eating and becomes withdrawn, holding his knees and not responding to a trusted friend, suspicion must be aroused that something is wrong. A process of elimination should remove factors such as constipation, diarrhoea, changes in medication or its side effects, tenderness of any areas of the body, major upsets in relationships, urinary tract infection and so on. Once the assessor is assured that nothing acutely obvious can be found, some hypotheses can be formed and tested by hot packs to the knees, paracetamol, rest, massage, comfort and reassurance. If the symptoms appear to be relieved by these measures, the chances of the pain being related to aching knees from arthritis increases. Observation will detect how often the person seems to have pain, what predisposes the behaviour and whether the intervention is actually improving the situation. Assessment and evaluation tools useful for assessing pain in older people are offered in Appendices 8.3 and 8.4.

Because of the difficulty of assessing older people with cognitive losses, direct observation may be the only way to establish the presence of pain. Observation of behaviour that suddenly alters for unidentifiable reasons may indicate the presence of pain. Appendix 8.5 offers an observation chart useful for assessing older people with impaired cognition.

abnormal tissue growth in older people

Changes in body defence mechanisms and the increased likelihood of exposure to carcinogens in the environment in ageing increases the chances of developing malignant changes in tissues in old age. Cancer is a change in body cells that transforms them into abnormal structures, capable of rapidly dividing and mutating so that the cell loses its correct function. The ability to migrate and cause secondary foci is also possible. Environmental factors include exposure to chemicals, smoke inhalation, coal and asbestos dust, and high ultraviolet sunrays.

Skin cancer remains the most common abnormal condition in older people. Changes in moles and pigmented areas exposed to the sun result in lesions. Lips, noses, ears and hands are the most common sites. The abnormal growth can be basal cell or squamous cell carcinoma. Melanoma occurs in the melanocyte cells and is noted for the dark discolouration and irregular outline of the lesion. Melanoma is the most likely metastatic forming cancer (Holmes, 1997).

Further information can be obtained from any branch of the Cancer Council and it is wise to obtain a coloured poster of the changes in cells to assist in differentiation. Initial changes are usually painless and can be mistaken for the changes in ageing skin. Any lesion that changes in shape or colour, discharges and/or becomes painful must be checked by an expert medical practitioner.

Seventy per cent of breast cancer occurs in women over 50, with many older women remaining undetected even though western countries have breast screening programs that include mammography. Unfortunately, older women frequently do not avail themselves of these programs in the misguided belief that they are immune because of age. Assessment of breast tissue for older women can be embarrassing and is not performed as routinely as for younger women. The risk factors increase for women who have a family history, have had other cancers, and who smoke. Inspection should be undertaken looking for symmetry between breasts, dimpling, wrinkled patches of indented skin or peau d'orange, discharge from nipples, nipple retraction or oedema. Palpation that reveals a hard, immobile lump in the breast tissue or lymph nodes should result in the person seeking immediate medical attention.

The treatment of breast cancer depends on the age and physical condition of the woman. A frail older woman may elect to have a lumpectomy and no further treatment. Further radiation or chemotherapy treatment can be effective and the decision remains with the person and their family.

In older males, the development of prostate cancer is relatively common. Benign prostate enlargement is easily treated by resection and similar removal of cancerous growth can be done in the early stages. Once the spread of carcinoma into the surrounding prostatic capsule occurs, metastatic spread to bone is common. A medical practitioner or health practitioner who has experience in rectal and abdominal palpation best performs assessment of older males' uro-genital systems. Any reduction in stream during micturition, painful urination, bladder distension and blood in the urine may be symptomatic and should be checked.

continuous quality improvement issues

In a residential care setting, the recording of any skin breakdown is imperative for quality assurance databanks to provide the information to monitor improvement in care. Predisposing factors in skin breakdown can be dealt with before further problems develop. Quality issues identified by examination of data may relate to poorly kept equipment, lack of staff education, lack of resources to properly manage wounds, inadequate nutrition, polypharmacy, over use of sedation, scratching with long fingernails by the person themselves, poor techniques in moving people, ill-fitting clothing and poor continence management. If any predisposing factor can be identified consistently, there should be a plan to rectify the problem and initiate ongoing evaluation.

case study: Mrs Drew

Mrs Drew was admitted to your care because she could no longer live alone at home. She was assessed as Category 5 for low-level care placement. On admission, she presented as a thin, pale and tearful lady with a grubby bandage on her left foot. Her weight was 52 kg and her blood pressure 190/100. Her left foot was unbandaged and an infected big toe was revealed. There was a large amount of offensive pus present. Swabs grew a MRSA (multiple resistant *Staphylococcus aureus*) and the infection seemed to be spreading into the web space between her toes.

case study questions

1   Would Mrs Drew's weight influence healing?
2   What do you understand about Mrs Drew's mental state, and would this influence healing?
3   How would you commence wound assessment on Mrs Drew?
4   Identify the major assessment strategies you would implement for Mrs Drew.

conclusion

Older people have special needs and observations are required to promote healing and to build immunity to protect tissues. The normal parameters of ageing predispose the body to have less than normal operating defence systems. Assessment must be thorough and undertaken with detailed observations and reliable assessment tools. The increased incidence of cancer in older people is also an important factor in the assessment process. Healing of damaged tissue is a most important issue in aged care and if not addressed by proper assessment, managed and evaluated correctly, the potential for complications of a systemic nature is very high.

study questions

1   What impact does stress have on the ageing body?
2   What observations should be made to determine the health status of the skin of an older person?
3   Breakdown in the integrity of the skin can be through tears, wounds and pressure or shearing forces. Explain the differences.
4   What factors predispose an older person to pressure ulcers?
5   Why are dependable recording tools important in care?
6   How should a continuous quality improvement program collect data, and for what reasons?

references

Braden, B. J. and Bergstrom, N. (1987), 'Clinical utility of the Braden Scale for predicting pressure sore risk', *Decubitus*, 2(3), pp. 44–51.

Carotenuto, R. and Bullock, J. (1981), *Physical Assessment of the Gerontologic Client*, F. A. Davis, Philadelphia.

Chandra, B. K. (1992), 'Effect of vitamin and trace element supplementation on immune responses and infection in elderly subjects', *Lancet*, 340, pp. 1124–7.

Ferguson, J. and MacLean, D. (1997), 'Wound management in older people', *The Australian Journal of Hospital Pharmacy*, Vol. 27, No. 6, pp. 461–7.

Groer, M. E. and Shekelton M. E. (1979), *Basic Pathophysiology: A Conceptual Approach*, C. V. Mosby, St Louis, Missouri.

Holmes, H. N. (ed.) (1997), *Mastering Geriatric Care*, Springhouse Corporation, Springhouse, Pennsylvania.

Lueckenotte, A. G. (ed.) (1996), *Gerontologic Nursing*, Mosby, St Louis, Missouri.

Appendix 8.1: Residential care services Skin integrity assessment

Name .... Resident ID no: .... Room no: ....
Signed .... Assessed on: ....

Past history
Pressure ulcer ....
Leg ulcers ....
Sensitivities ....
Other ....
....

Health status
☐ Diabetic   ☐ Poor circulation   ☐ Poor nutrition
Other
(comment) ....

☐ Obese   ☐ Thin

Oedema   ☐ Yes   ☐ No
Type ....
Area ....

☐ Incontinent urine   ☐ Incontinent faeces

☐ Chair fast   ☐ Bed fast   ☐ Limited mobility

Dry skin
☐ Arms   ☐ Legs   ☐ Face   ☐ Torso

Tissue-paper skin
☐ Arms   ☐ Legs   ☐ Torso
Other
(comment) ....

Excoriation or reddened areas
☐ Groin   ☐ Abdominal flap   ☐ Under breasts
☐ Axilla   ☐ Neck   ☐ Hands
Other
(comment) ....

Rash or allergies
☐ Arms   ☐ Legs   ☐ Torso   ☐ Face
(describe) ....
....

Appendix 8.1: (continued)

Bruises
☐ Arms ☐ Legs ☐ Torso
Other
(comment) ....

Show bruises, wounds, scars, excoriations, rashes, skin tears on diagram

Hair
☐ Stringy ☐ Dull ☐ Dry
☐ Lustrous ☐ Shiny

Condition of scalp
☐ Healthy ☐ Dry ☐ Scaly
☐ Other

(comment) ....

Nails

Fingernails	☐ Ingrown	☐ Overgrown	☐ Thickened
	☐ Brittle	☐ Discoloured	☐ Corns or callouses
Toenails	☐ Ingrown	☐ Overgrown	☐ Thickened
	☐ Brittle	☐ Discoloured	☐ Corns or callouses
	☐ Overlapping	☐ Hammer toe	☐ Hallus valuges

Appendix 8.2: Residential care services Wound assessment and progress chart

Surname: .... Given name: .... Room no: ....

Signed: .... Designation: .... Date: ....

Diabetes: YES   NO
State type & management: ....
Smoker: YES   NO
Respiratory illness: YES   NO
Anaemia: YES   NO
Nutritional status (eg, poor appetite, underweight, nil orally): ....
....

Type of wound (describe): ....
....
Duration of wound: ....

Quality of surrounding skin
    Inflamed   Macerated   Friable   Dry   Crusty   Fragile

    Other (state): ....

Wound microbiology:

Swab taken: YES   NO   If yes, date taken: ....
Result: ....

Sensitivities: ....

Antibiotics required: YES   NO   If yes, type & dosage: ....

Dressings

Date	Cleansing agent	Dressing product	Bandage	Frequency

Appendix 8.2: (continued)

Location (detail on diagram)

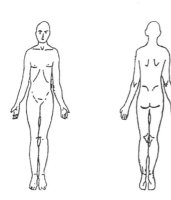

Colour of wound Record % of wound surface that is covered by the corresponding colour B Black Y Yellow R Red	Volume of exudate N None S Small M Moderate H Heavy

Wound depth score

Score	Description
1	superficial/epidermal layer
2	extending to dermal layer
3	extending to subcutaneous layer
4	extending to muscle/tendon/bone
5	extending to compartments

Review date					
Dimension (draw wound & show measurement) A ↔ cm B ↑ cm					
Depth score					
Colour					
Volume of exudate					
Sign & date					
Review date					
Dimension (draw wound & show measurement) A ↔ cm B ↑ cm					
Depth score					
Colour					
Volume of exudate					
Sign & date					
Review date					
Dimension (draw wound & show measurement) A ↔ cm B ↑ cm					
Depth score					
Colour					
Volume of exudate					
Sign & date					

Appendix 8.3: Residential care services Pain assessment chart

Surname: .... Given name: ....
Resident ID no: .... Room no: ....

Manner of expressing pain: Verbal   Resident's description (prick, ache, burn, throb etc) ....
....
                                 Non-verbal cues   Describe non-verbal cues
....
....

Onset & duration: ....

Effects of pain: (Note decreased function, decreased quality of life and accompanying symptoms; eg, nausea)

Sleep: ....

Appetite: ....

Physical activity: ....
....

Relationship with others (eg, irritability): ....

Emotions (eg, anger, fear, crying, depression): ....

Other: ....
....

What causes or makes the pain(s) worse? ....
....
....

What helps to relieve the pain(s)? ....
....
....

Appendix 8.3: (continued)

Pain sites (mark pain sites on diagram)

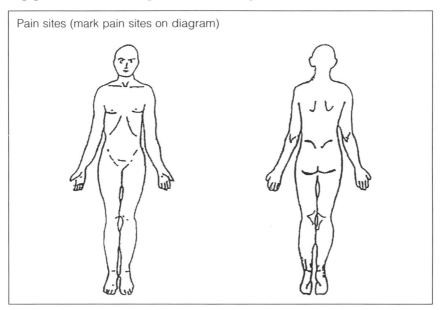

Pain management plan to be developed from data gathered from pain assessment form and pain assessment chart

Pain management plan (to be added to resident care plan)

....
....
....
....
....
....
....
....
....
....
....
....
....
....
....
....
....

Name of assessor: ....
Signature: ....
Date: ....

Reproduced with permission, Vision Australia Foundation

Appendix 8.4: Residential services Pain management evaluation chart

| Surname: .... Given names: .... Resident no: .... |
| Date of assessment: .... Signed: .... |

Key to pain intensity	Possible pain behaviours
0 No pain	Noisy breathing
1–2 Mild pain	Negative vocalisation
3–4 Moderate pain	Sad facial expression
5–6 Severe pain	Frightened facial expression
7–8 Very severe pain	Frown
9–10 Overwhelming pain	Tense body language
S Sleep	Brow lowering
	Fidgeting

Comments can include: activity, position of comfort, other pain relief measures, contributing or related factors and side effects such as bowel function, nausea, vomiting.

Date & time	Area & intensity Possible pain behaviour	Intervention/analgesia Comments on effectiveness

Appendix 8.5: Residential care services Pain observation chart for cognitively impaired resident

Surname: .... Given name: .... Resident ID NO: ....
Date of assessment: .... Signed: ....

This chart is to be used when observing the possibility of pain for a resident who cannot express their feelings verbally. The purpose is to link the behaviour thought to be an expression of pain with the response to therapy/intervention or analgesia. The behaviour is noted and observed over a period of one week (or longer if required) and the response to any intervention is recorded and implemented consistently to gauge responses.

Date & time	Possible pain behaviour	Strategy tried	Comments on effectiveness

Reproduced with permission, Vision Australia Foundation

assessment of fluid dynamics and common symptoms of imbalance

Sally Garratt

chapter summary

This chapter outlines the interrelationships that exist between the major fluid systems in the ageing body and the physiological responses to altered composition and shifts of these fluids. Maintaining a balanced state between the intracellular and extracellular fluid compartments is essential for health and wellbeing. Ageing cells are more susceptible to damage; therefore, ionic changes and fluid shifts can lead to sudden and rapid health deterioration. Symptoms of impending trouble can be mistakenly attributed to normal ageing rather than important subtle changes from pathological events. The development of oedema, dehydration and renal malfunction are discussed, with strategies for assessing the fluid and ionic balance status of the older person.

objectives

After reading and reflecting on this chapter, you will be able to:

- identify the major fluid compartments of the body and predominant ions
- discuss the reasons for fluid shifts
- describe the reasons for oedema
- describe the implications of imbalance due to hypoxia
- identify the potential for imbalance due to diabetes mellitus
- examine the strategies for assessment of states of imbalance
- discuss the importance of identifying older people at risk and employing preventative action
- identify symptoms indicating the need for emergency attention.

introduction

Assessment of the fluid and electrolyte (ionic) balance of an older person is an important part of any comprehensive data gathering process. Actual states of imbalance may not be present at the time of initial assessment; however, the potential for an imbalance to occur must be determined and strategies to circumvent potential problems should be considered and implemented. Risk factors can be assessed and should be recorded in the nursing notes if the risk is determined to be significant. The eight-step problem-solving model in Chapter 1 illustrates the need for hypotheses for testing that will assist in determining risk.

Fluid and electrolyte replacement programs can be introduced, if necessary, before the danger signals of major malfunction begin. Conversely, a reduction in fluid intake or accelerating fluid loss may be necessary in some cases. Skilled nursing assessment is not difficult if the process is undertaken systematically to establish a baseline from which changes in fluid dynamics could be determined and decisions can be made. Once a baseline has been recorded, deviations from this are more easily identified if problems arise or subtle changes are discovered six months later.

what are the fluid compartments of interest?

The ageing body reacts to changes in fluid shifts very quickly. Any alterations in the fluid volumes of the cells (intracellular compartment), interstitial spaces (extracellular compartment) or vessels (blood/plasma) also results in disturbance of the ionic balance and vice versa. Life-threatening situations can occur. The major ions, or electrolytes, are potassium, chloride, sodium and calcium; other ions are bicarbonate, magnesium, sulphate and phosphate. The plasma also carries other trace elements such as zinc. Electrolyte levels are regulated through the action of hormones and kidney function.

Since 40 per cent of total body weight is made up of intracellular fluid (approximately 25 litres), 15 per cent in the extracellular compartment and 5 per cent in blood, any shift of fluid towards the outside of the cell into extracellular space will cause observable signs. Any reduction in total body water will take longer to be demonstrated as the body compensates by drawing fluid from the cells and interstitial spaces towards the vessels to maintain the flow of nutrients and oxygen as long as possible (Vander et al., 1986).

The fluid in each compartment has a distinct electrolyte balance. The intracellular compartment fluid has more potassium, phosphate and protein, while the extracellular fluid compartment has more sodium and chloride. Cell membranes are freely permeable to water and usually impermeable to protein and other colloids. The movement of electrolytes is selective and accomplished by both active and passive processes. Osmosis, diffusion and filtration are the passive ways in which water and electrolytes move across cell membranes. Concentrations of the major ions rising or falling in any of the fluid compartments will cause water to shift by osmosis, or from the area of low concentration towards the area of higher concentration. Osmotic pull will continue to occur until equilibrium is reached. Reading a physiology text will help you to understand the full mechanisms of this process. This chapter aims simply to demonstrate how fluid shifts can be observed and to assist the assessor to know when to take action.

The concentration of ions and also the amount of plasma proteins or colloids present affects fluid composition in the vessels. The large plasma protein molecules prevent leakage of water at the capillary level by balancing the osmotic forces between the plasma and the interstitial water concentration. Normally a very small filtration of water into the interstitial spaces is picked up and returned by the lymphatic system. The lymphatic system is the only way proteins that escape from the intravascular compartment can be returned to the plasma. From this very brief overview, we can begin to explore the common symptoms of fluid imbalance that nurses observe in older people. The most often observed and reported symptom is oedema.

oedema

Oedema is due to an excess of fluid in the extracellular space or interstitial tissues. Why should this occur? Consider the factors that influence fluid shifts:

- the hydrostatic pressure in the vessels changes
- the composition of the fluid in the compartments changes
- the tissue and/or vessels are damaged by external trauma.

changes in vessel pressures

Alterations in circulatory pressures occur because of changes to the pump, changes to the vessel walls, or changes in the blood. The pump, or heart, may begin to fail in older people. Heart muscle can be affected by infarction, valve disease and decreased contractility. Poor contraction leads to poor cardiac output and a general slowing of the circulation. Initially, the heart compensates by dilatation and lengthening of the myocardial muscle fibres. An enlarged heart requires more blood flow to sustain the muscle and as the rate of enlargement is not compensated for by the production of more vessels to supply the muscle fast enough, the end result is a slowing of the heart contractility (Groer and Shekleton, 1979). The collection of symptoms of decreased energy, shortness of breath and peripheral oedema is categorised as congestive cardiac failure. The slowing heart becomes engorged with a backlog of blood, venous return is slowed and the capillary bed becomes congested with increased plasma volume (Vander et al., 1986). Water shifts into the tissues and swelling occurs. The fluid is influenced by gravity and tends to pool in the lower extremities. When oedema occurs over the tibia and light pressure from a finger causes an indentation or pit in the tissue, the term 'pitting' oedema is used. Pitting can also be elicited over the sacrum, sternum or fibula.

At the same time as observable tissue swelling occurs, other organs are also becoming congested. The air sacs of the lungs can also fill with fluid due to increased pulmonary capillary pressure, causing the life-threatening situation of pulmonary oedema. When fluid accumulates in the alveoli, the ability to exchange gases is affected. Oxygenation of the blood falls below normal and the respiratory centre accelerates the rate of respiration to compensate. Hypoxia affects all tissues and the brain is affected immediately with ensuing confusion, delirium and eventually coma. The kidneys also suffer from renal congestion and excrete excessive amounts of potassium and the subsequent failure of sodium and water excretion compounds the problem (Holmes, 1997).

Hormonal alterations, nervous system baroreceptor interference and hypertension can bring about changes to the blood vessels themselves. Hypertension or high blood pressure is usually related to abnormally constricted arterioles, leading to increased peripheral resistance. In other words, the heart is pumping harder to get blood through narrower vessels. Hormones can influence the diameter or blood vessels (eg, adrenalin secreted in response to fright, or epinephrine from tumours of the renal medulla). Atheroma and arteriosclerosis can affect the walls of arteries and arterioles. Hardening of the vessel walls is due to thickening of connective tissue and deposits of cholesterol accumulating over time. This problem is predominantly lifestyle related and is most often referred to as a disease of ageing. Wherever the problem occurs, there is a change in the blood flow and pressure within the vessel alters.

Venous pressure is increased in obstruction from thrombosis and usually affects the calf, with lower limb oedema as a result. Oedema of the upper limb is usually the result of lymphatic obstruction causing accumulation of protein in the interstitial space (Vardaxis, 1994).

changes in fluid composition

Changes in the composition of the fluid in compartments is usually linked to the movement of water through sodium shifts and resultant hydrostatic pressure changes at the capillary beds. As sodium is the principal cation of the extracellular fluid, it largely determines the volume of that compartment. Too much sodium will lead to circulatory congestion and pulmonary oedema. A lack of sodium will lead to volume depletion and circulatory shock. A sodium deficit can result from reduced intake or excessive loss, usually from the gastrointestinal tract. Normally sodium is absorbed from the colon but in cases of diarrhoea, the increased motility does not allow this to happen. Sodium is also lost in sweat; however, excessive sweating is not common in older people without sustained pathological problems. Heat exhaustion can induce loss of water and sodium in sweat and if both are not replaced, the result is hypotonic contraction of the body fluid. If this condition progresses to heat stroke, the sweating stops and body temperature continues to rise, leading to cell death, coma and death. Alteration in plasma protein can be due to a lack of protein in the diet, a reduction in the synthesis of plasma proteins by the liver or nephrotic syndrome where the kidneys excrete protein.

Medication use can also play a large role in the alteration of body fluids and electrolytes. Diuretics, corticosteroids, hormone replacements, antihypertensives, prolonged use of antacids or purgatives, and some antibiotics can alter the absorption and balance of ions and water.

tissue or vessel trauma

Trauma to tissue from burns, severe bruising, lacerations and allergic reactions can also cause a shift in plasma proteins with resultant changes in interstitial pressures and development of oedema. This form of oedema is hard or 'brawny', the tissue is tight with no pitting and swelling remains localised. Lymphatic obstruction from removal of axillary lymph nodes during mastectomy often causes this form of oedema in the affected arm. Allergic reactions in the throat or larynx can be life-threatening as airways close with the swelling and hypoxia results. If oedema occurs in the brain, through either trauma or disease, the intracranial pressure increases and signs of cerebral distress are manifested in alterations in consciousness, irregular pupillary reactions, paralysis, vomiting, headache, depressed respiration, decreased pulse rate and increased blood pressure. Older people who sustain cerebral haemorrhage can exhibit signs of cerebral oedema and require urgent emergency intervention.

The major concern for long-term care of older people is when lesions occur; where there is oedematous tissue there is a reduction in healing. Oedmatous tissue is prone to breakdown and more susceptible to infection. Lower extremities are more likely to be traumatised through walking into objects or simply scratching the skin, exposing the tissue to the development of infection and/or ulceration. Oedema precludes efficient delivery of oxygen and nutrients to the cells and hypoxia with acidosis will follow, impeding healing.

Clinicians also need to be aware of the 'third space' syndrome. This occurs when a large amount of extracellular fluid remains in the body in a particular area and is unavailable to the effective circulation. Fluid build-up in body cavities through such trauma as intestinal obstruction, major vessel obstruction in the thorax or abdomen, crushing injuries, bleeding into a cavity, peritonitis, metastatic fluid or ascites can be insidious or develop rapidly. Rapid fluid shifts result in tachycardia and hypotension and require urgent attention.

dehydration: why are older people prone to dehydration?

A normal healthy adult will maintain fluid and electrolyte balance through the physiological mechanisms mediated by hormones, mainly antidiuretic hormone and aldosterone, through receptor stimulation and renal regulation. The phenomenon of thirst, defined as 'the conscious desire for water' (Guyton, 1979), is the primary regulator for the intake of water. The control mechanisms are so tight we cannot overindulge in water intake, we simply excrete it through the kidneys until balance is

reached. Whenever we are lacking in water, the thirst centre of the hypo-
thalamus triggers the immediate need to drink. In older people, this
thirst trigger may be impaired, the renal system may not be as efficient,
and water and sodium balance regulation slows or is not detected as
rapidly. Losses can therefore be severe before the osmoreceptor sites are
stimulated to conserve or demand water.

Other factors involved in the ability to increase intake of water
are impaired mobility to actually get a drink, cognitive loss that impairs
the ability to request fluid, the type of fluid available (as most older
people have traditionally favoured tea or other fluids rather than
water), and medication that sedates or impairs swallowing or desire for
fluid. Depression is not uncommon in older people and the desire to be
left alone can outweigh the need for fluid. Psychological factors may
include the notion that increased fluid intake impairs continence and
that asking for something to drink is being a nuisance for staff. The use
of diuretics can also influence sodium and potassium loss and fluid
balance.

acid–base balance

Maintaining the acid–base balance means regulation of the hydrogen ion
concentration in body fluids. The normal concentration of hydrogen ions
keeps the pH of arterial blood at 7.4 and venous blood at 7.35 because
of extra carbon dioxide. Acidosis occurs when the pH falls below these
values and alkalosis when the pH rises above them. Poor blood flow to
any tissue causes carbon dioxide accumulation and a decrease in pH
(Guyton, 1979). The normal defence mechanisms to maintain pH are the
acid–base buffer systems of bicarbonate, phosphate and proteins. The
major clinical abnormalities of acid–base balance are due to problems
with the respiratory system or problems with metabolism.

respiratory acidosis and alkalosis

Respiratory acidosis is caused by any factor that decreases the rate
and/or depth of ventilation, thus increasing the concentration of dis-
solved carbon dioxide in the extracellular fluid. This higher concentration leads to carbonic acid and hydrogen ions, thus resulting in acidosis.
Over-breathing, such as evidenced in forms of hysteria, leads to the
reverse situation of respiratory alkalosis, as too much carbon dioxide is
washed out. Pathologic conditions such as chronic obstructive airways
disease (COAD), damage to the respiratory centre in the medulla oblon-

gata, reduced surface in the alveoli such as fluid from pneumonia, collapsed lung or pneumothorax will cause acidosis. In chronic lung conditions, the carbon dioxide level is higher than normal and the carotid and aortic bodies' receptor sites become attuned to this. Too much oxygen will cause these receptors to cease responding and ventilation ceases. Other factors that influence the respiratory centre are temperature, pain, emotion, release of epinephrine, reflexes from joints and muscles, especially during exercise, and voluntary control of breathing (Vander et al., 1986).

metabolic acidosis

Metabolic acidosis can be the result of kidney failure, too much metabolic acid formed in the body, ingestion of acids, loss of alkalis from the body fluids and intravenous administration of metabolic acids. The most common forms of metabolic acidosis in older people is from diabetes mellitus, diarrhoea, vomiting, uremia and high extracellular fluid concentration of potassium. Severe diarrhoea in older people can be devastating, as large amounts of bicarbonate are lost from the intestinal fluid very quickly and the ability to maintain balance with hydrogen ions is compromised. Severe prolonged vomiting by itself is not common but in conjunction with diarrhoea the effects of bicarbonate loss are even more dramatic.

Uremic acidosis is found in severe renal disease where the kidneys cannot excrete the normal amounts of metabolic acid waste. Renal failure is evident when there is generalised oedema from water and sodium retention and high concentration of other urinary retention products such as creatinine, uric acid, phenols, sulphates, phosphates and potassium (Guyton, 1979). The severity of high concentrations of these waste products, especially those from protein catabolism, forming urea, can lead to coma and death.

diabetes mellitus

Diabetes mellitus produces a relative or absolute lack of insulin from the pancreas, leading to the prevention of glucose uptake by the cells. Instead, stored fats are catabolised for energy and the by-products of acetoacetic acid or ketones are released into the bloodstream. The kidneys excrete some of this, along with extra water, but accumulation in the blood leads to metabolic acidosis. The recognition of altered blood glucose levels is extremely important in the assessment of older people.

Prolonged high blood glucose leads to severe damage in many areas of the body (eg, the kidneys can develop diabetic nephropathy, there can be atherosclerosis of the blood vessels, hypercholesterolaemia, hypertension, myocardial infarction, arterial sclerosis of the lower limbs, liver fatty changes, diabetic retinopathy and slow cataracts in the eyes, trophic changes in the skin, increased susceptibility to infection in the lungs, sensory and motor neuropathy, boils and fungal infections and peripheral neuritis).

diagnostic criteria

The first criterion is a random venous plasma glucose greater than 11.1 mmol/L. This should be confirmed by a fasting plasma glucose equal to or greater than 7.0 mmol/L. Gluco-urinalysis is not effective as a diagnostic or monitoring aid in older people due to their having a higher renal threshold which may be up to 15–18 mmol/L or more (Dargarville, 1995). A more reliable test is a fasting blood glucose tolerance challenge.

glycaemic emergencies

Hypoglycaemia   Although some people may experience symptoms at higher levels, this condition is usually defined as a blood glucose level below 3.5 mmol/L. At this level, the symptoms of an insulin reaction or 'hypo' may become apparent and, if the blood glucose level is allowed to drop below 4 mmol/L, the diabetic person is at risk. Hypoglycaemia does not usually occur in diet-controlled diabetics but anyone being treated with tablets or insulin is at risk of becoming 'hypo'.

Signs and symptoms include:

- the sudden onset of internal feelings of unease or unwellness
- trembling
- sweating
- ravenous hunger
- palpitation of the heart
- headache
- tingling in the fingers and lips
- disturbances of concentration
- disorders of speech and sight
- aggressive behaviour
- confusion.

Diabetics may often sleep through 'hypos' that occur at night and the symptoms go unnoticed. However, the following signs may indicate unnoticed nocturnal hypoglycaemia:

- morning headaches
- 'hangover'
- sweaty nightwear
- pre-breakfast hyperglycaemia (Somogyi effect).

Likely causes of hypoglycaemia:

- missing a meal or insufficient carbohydrate intake
- exceptional physical stress without preventative measures
- inappropriate dose or accidental over-administration of insulin or tablets
- reduction in diet
- excessive alcohol intake
- intramuscular or intravenous injection of insulin
- vomiting (eg, morning sickness, gastroenteritis).

Treatment of early signs and symptoms:

- Immediate treatment is necessary. (Note: Hypoglycaemic episodes treated immediately are not known to cause any long lasting side effects.)
- Initially, some form of quickly absorbed carbohydrate should be given such as barely sugar, jelly beans, orange juice or soft drinks (not low calorie). Some form of sugar or sweetened drinks should be kept on the bedside table for emergencies (eg, hypos at night), since the diabetic may lapse into a hypoglycaemic coma (shock) if the early 'hypo' signs are not recognised and treated. This may lead to loss of consciousness and occasionally to fitting.
- A portion of carbohydrate such as a sandwich or a couple of biscuits and some cheese should follow this unless the 'hypo' occurs within 15 minutes of the next meal.
- The possible cause of the 'hypo' should be determined.
- A diabetic person who is treated with insulin or oral therapy should always carry some form of quickly absorbed carbohydrate.
- If the 'hypo' is severe and there is loss of consciousness, the unconscious person should be turned on her or his side and the airway checked and cleared if necessary.

- A medical order for glucagon 1–2 mg should be obtained and injected intramuscularly.
- If the diabetic person does not respond to the glucagon within 10 minutes, an ambulance must be called. Recovery will be hastened by the use of a 50 per cent solution of intravenous dextrose.
- If consciousness is restored by glucagon, glucose or sugar should be given by mouth followed by some food (eg, a sandwich) as soon as the person is able to swallow.
- Nothing to eat or drink should be given if a person is unable to swallow or is unconscious.

Hyperglycaemia   This is defined as a blood glucose level above the normal range (4–7 mmol/L). However, symptoms usually occur when blood glucose levels are greater than 15 mmol/L. Blood glucose levels persistently above 10 mmol/L increase the risk of long-term complications. If signs and symptoms associated with this higher level of blood glucose are left untreated, this can lead to vomiting and dehydration, alteration in consciousness and ketoacidosis in Type I diabetics. However, even mild elevations of blood glucose need to be corrected in order to minimise the development of long-term complications. Type I diabetes is also referred to as insulin-dependent diabetes mellitus (IDDM).

Signs and symptoms of excessively high blood glucose are:

- excessive urination
- increased thirst
- tiredness
- weight loss
- recurrent infections (eg, pruritus vulvae, balanitis, skin infections).

Note: Some diabetics, in particular those with Type II diabetes, may have blood glucose levels greater than 15 mmol/L without experiencing these symptoms.—Type II diabetes is also referred to as non–insulin-dependent diabetes mellitus (NIDDM).

Likely causes of hyperglycaemia:

- excessive carbohydrate intake
- prolonged reduction of usual physical activity
- inadvertent injection of too little insulin or forgetting the injection
- omission of tablets (Type II diabetes)
- infection

- stress
- rebound after hypoglycaemia (Somogyi effect)
- other medications (eg, steroids)
- menstruation
- pregnancy.

Note: If the blood glucose is persistently above 15 mmol/L, particularly if this is due to a prolonged illness such as influenza or measles, extra insulin is required and the person's medical officer must be notified. The following treatment will be required:

- Injections of short-acting insulin will be required in addition to the usual dose of long-acting insulin.
- The short-acting insulin should be injected every hour until the blood glucose falls below 10 mmol/L.
- The suggested dose of short-acting insulin is 2–4 units for children and 4–6 units for adults.
- It is important to continue the usual carbohydrate intake while the extra insulin is being taken. This can be taken in liquid form if the person is unable to eat.
- One cup of fluid should be taken every hour.

Prolonged vomiting may also cause blood glucose levels above 15 mmol/L and increases in urinary ketones. Vomiting may be caused by:

- gastric infection
- migraine
- intolerance to antibiotics or other drugs
- sometimes after severe hypoglycaemia
- morning sickness during pregnancy.

  If vomiting does occur:

- the usual insulin dose should always be given
- the usual carbohydrate intake should be consumed (if necessary, fluids equivalent in carbohydrate content can be substituted for foods)
- hourly tests for blood glucose and urine ketones should be done
- it is preferable to avoid the use of anti-vomiting medicines, some of which may cause drowsiness at a time when alertness is desirable

- if blood glucose is less than 10 mmol/L, ordinary flat lemonade should be taken until the vomiting subsides—about a third of a glass every 20 minutes.

Note: If, as a result of prolonged vomiting, the blood glucose is above 15 mmol/L with moderate to large ketones in the urine, a doctor should be called at once. This indicates the threatening metabolic crisis of ketoacidosis, requiring immediate medical attention.

Ketoacidosis This condition is usually restricted to Type I diabetes and is defined as severe hyperglycaemia accompanied by the accumulation of moderate to large amounts of ketones in the urine. Ketones are acids that alter the normal acid–base balance of the body, and therefore ketoacidosis is considered a medical emergency requiring immediate medical treatment.

Possible precipitating causes:

- an intercurrent illness
- vomiting
- omission or reduction of insulin dose
- a prolonged period of neglect of usual diabetes treatment
- stress.

Testing for urinary ketones is essential during periods of illness and/or vomiting and during episodes of severe hyperglycaemia if ketoacidosis to be averted. Signs of ketoacidosis are as follows:

- onset over some hours
- thirst and polyuria
- dehydration
- nausea and/or vomiting
- weakness of muscles
- abdominal pain
- drowsiness, coma
- Kussmaul respirations
- acetone breath
- hypotension
- tachycardia
- hypothermia
- ketonuria and hyperglycaemia.

Elderly people who have Type II diabetes also have the potential for hyperglycaemic, hyperosmolar, non-ketotic syndrome. This condition requires urgent medical intervention and is manifested by:

- drowsiness
- confusion
- hypotension
- onset over days or longer
- no ketones
- not acidotic
- infection present
- an elevated white cell count
- osmolality (> 330 mOsm/L)

(Protocols reproduced with permission of Vision Australia Foundation—Bridget Quigley.)

action of diuretics in acid–base balance

Diuretics are substances that increase the rate of urine output. They can do this in two main ways, either by increasing the glomerular filtration rate or by decreasing the rate of fluid reabsorption from the tubules. Digitalis, theophylline, caffeine and norepinephrine will influence the glomerular filtration rate and increase fluid loss. These are weak diuretics and can only increase the rate or urinary output two- to four-fold (Guyton, 1979).

Osmotic diuretics, such as mannitol, sucrose or urea, act on the tubules by increasing osmotic pressure, thus causing large amounts of water to flush through. Diabetes mellitus causes the same effect, as high blood sugar acts as an osmotic force causing high urine output. Furosemide and ethacrynic acid are the most powerful agents for diuresis. They act on the loop of Henle and block the absorption of sodium and chloride ions, causing, under acute conditions, urine outputs as great as 25 times normal. Their action is short lived but the effect is rapid and effective. The thiazide diuretics act on the distal tubules and cortical portions of the collecting tubules to prevent active sodium reabsorption (Guyton, 1979). Acetazolamide blocks reabsorption of bicarbonate ions from the proximal tubules and can lead to a degree of acidosis because of the loss of bicarbonate from body fluids. Spironolactone blocks the effects of aldosterone, thus blocking sodium reabsorption. Alcohol, hypnotics, anaesthetics and narcotics inhibit anti-diuretic hormone secretion and cause increased urinary output.

metabolic alkalosis

This condition is not common but can occur through the use of some diuretics, the excessive ingestion of alkaline drugs for stomach acidity, loss of chloride ions through vomiting and reducing gastric acids, and excessive aldosterone production by the adrenal glands. The major effect of alkalosis on the body is excitability of the central nervous system, leading to confusion and coma. One of the diagnostic signs of metabolic alkalosis is decreased pulmonary ventilation. Conversely, the rate of ventilation is increased in respiratory acidosis, as this is the cause of the problem. Alkalosis is manifested in overexcitability of the nervous system with tetanic spasms of muscles, leading to tetany of the respiratory muscles and death.

hypoxia

Hypoxia is a reduction in oxygen at the tissue level. Ischemic hypoxia results from insufficient blood flow to the tissues; histotoxic hypoxia results from a toxic agent interfering with the ability of the cells to use oxygen; anaemic hypoxia is due to a lack of haemoglobin in the red cells, reducing their oxygen carrying capacity; and hypoxic hypoxia occurs where there is a reduction of arterial oxygen. Older people are at greater risk of hypoxia because of their fragile ability to regain balance quickly in response to factors impinging on their health. Ischemic hypoxia is common in the extremities because of insufficient cardiac output, and histotoxic hypoxia may be evident following anaesthesia or other drug therapy.

assessment of risk factors for fluid and electrolyte imbalance in older people

Any older person who has a previous history of, or is presenting with, any of the following symptoms should be considered to be at risk and monitored closely.

sudden increase in body weight with uncomfortable feeling

This may be due to fluid retention or ascities formation. Fluid in the lower extremities, especially pitting, together with difficulty in breathing suggests fluid in the pulmonary system and cardiac failure. Ascities, or fluid in the abdominal cavity, may be present from malignant growth or bowel obstruction and peritonitis.

abnormal urine testing

Abnormal urine testing (ie, altered pH, specific gravity, presence of protein or blood) suggests renal disease such as chronic nephritis or infection and may also reflect diabetes mellitus, tumours, starvation, or liver disease. Multistix routine testing is useful for screening purposes but laboratory testing is essential for confirming diagnosis.

cardiac problems

Oedema of the extremities, headache, rapid pulse, known cardiac output problems, and medication such as digoxin, diuretics or antihypertensives suggest chronic circulatory disease (eg, tachycardia, hypertension).

respiratory problems

Symptoms such as dyspnoea, orthopnoea, or paroxysmal nocturnal dyspnoea are serious indicators of respiratory disease and impending pulmonary oedema and/or hypoxia. Caution in the administration of oxygen is necessary in chronic respiratory conditions.

altered blood gases

Altered blood gases (ie, high or low CO_2 or PCO_2 suggest either respiratory or metabolic acidosis alkalosis and require immediate further investigation.

known disease processes

Obvious pathological processes (eg, ulcerative colitis, kidney disease, respiratory diseases, diabetes mellitus, brain tumours, abdominal obstruction, altered hormonal states) that affect the ability to balance fluid and electrolytes should be monitored, and baseline blood gases and biochemical values plus observations are essential to identify the progress of the disease.

past episode of heat stroke in summer

Older people react to heat, and their temperature control mechanisms are often impaired by other cerebral problems. The ability to respond to heat in summer may be slower or not as visible as in younger adults. The sweating and thirst mechanisms are often impaired. If the person has had problems with temperature control in the past, they are at higher risk for further heat stroke.

medication

Prolonged use of medication (eg, constant use of diuretics, antacids, steroids or antihypertensives) without adequate monitoring can lead to overdose and shifts in renal control of absorption or excretion of electrolytes. The use of potassium supplements with some diuretics is common, but regular screening of blood levels of cortisol, digoxin, electrolytes and albumin is rarely done properly in older people.

repeated infections or high fever

Any infective process that causes fluid loss (eg, viral or bacterial diarrhoea, or ulcers) has the potential for acid–base balance shifts. Repeated chronic infections such as fungus or of nosocomial causation may be due to impaired immune responses or high blood glucose levels.

swallowing difficulties through cerebrovascular impairment

Cerebrovascular accident or repeated transient ischaemic attacks (TIAs) may affect the cranial nerves or motor pathways to impede swallowing. Parental feeding or percutaneous endoscopic gastroscopy (PEG) feeding systems may also lead to an excessive protein intake without sufficient water to flush the metabolic waste from the renal system. Uraemia is a dangerous condition that requires immediate attention.

poor nutrition and inadequate protein intake

Many older people who live alone do not consider their nutrition, or cannot afford to purchase fresh food and suffer from a lack of daily protein and vitamins. The resultant alteration in plasma albumin alters the fluid pressure dynamics in the blood vessels and fluid shifts occur.

persistent headache and change in concentration or awareness

Any altered level of consciousness and coherence must be fully investigated. Headache can suggest intra-cerebral pressure changes and the resultant impact on the pituitary or other key centres of the brain will lead to fluid and electrolyte shifts.

gastrointestinal changes, diarrhoea, vomiting, excessive thirst

Excessive thirst is rare in older adults and would suggest diabetes insipidus or severe acid–base disturbance. Diarrhoea and vomiting is easily observable and must be monitored carefully during any attack. Major acid–base disturbance can occur within a very short time if large amounts of fluid are lost.

pain that precludes eating and drinking

Older people are often stoic about pain and the refusal of fluids or food can be mistakenly attributed to behavioural attention seeking, lack of appetite or enthusiasm for eating with others, lack of taste buds or sensory stimulation and disliked foods. Long-term chronic pain from arthritis or ulceration of lower limbs can be overlooked as a contributing factor in nutrition. Astute observation is necessary to detect changes in expression, immobility or unusual behaviour indicative of pain, especially in older people who have dementia.

muscle twitching and hypertonicity, tetany or spasms

Prolonged use of antacids or other medications that alter the ability to match acid to base may be present. Lack of serum calcium can cause tetanic spasms in muscles and is very painful. Convulsions may develop and also respiratory failure.

falls and trauma such as fractured ribs, fistulas and burns

Haemorrhage into the tissues or body cavities from trauma, fracture sites and bruising can cause fluid shifts and resultant acid–base problems. Fractures of large bones and hip joints have the potential for serious blood loss into the surrounding tissues. Continuous drainage from a large fistula (eg, between the bowel and abdominal surface) can cause major loss of fluid and electrolytes. Burns and scalds cause protein and fluid loss into blisters and oozing tissue. Trauma is obviously easily recognised and commencing appropriate treatment with pain relief should preclude hypovolaemic shock developing (Hamilton, 1982).

the effects of immobility

Older people may have impaired mobility for many reasons. Often, joint and bone conditions such as arthritis and osteoporosis cause pain on movement and lead to a reduction in motor activity. Sensory loss and unfamiliar surroundings can preclude the ability to exercise and sedation or psychotropic medication may also inhibit movement. The prolonged use of restraint, either physical or chemical, may lead to the eventual inability to move, as joints and muscles stiffen and metabolic changes occur. Loss of endurance is related to the atrophy of muscles and is a cyclic phenomenon that creates a downward spiral. The more the muscles atrophy, the less endurance the person has and the less likely it is that they are able to move the muscles to prevent further atrophy.

Weakness due to atrophy of muscle and general slowing of the metabolic rate affects stability, and if the posture is such that muscle fibres are shortened by flexion, contractures may develop. Foot drop is also a factor in muscle stretching and tendon fibrosis from immobility and a reduction in bone mass, or osteoporosis, is also a concern. If this condition is severe enough, pathological fractures will occur and movement becomes more restricted. Immobility also leads to impaired oxygenation processes. There is a reduction in red blood cells, thus reducing the oxygen carrying capacity; poorer chest and lung expansion that accelerates hypostatic pneumonia; and increased chances of forming thrombus or emboli.

The chemical imbalances that occur through immobility include a negative calcium balance, negative nitrogen balance, and a compartmental fluid shift in dependent areas (Groer and Shekleton, 1979). Bladder and digestive tract disturbance are also contributing factors as water will be reabsorbed from the gut and resultant constipation begins a cycle of pressure alterations that increases the risk of circulatory problems. Immobility is therefore something to be avoided with older people and walking or exercise of some form is essential on a daily basis to prevent the serious consequences developing.

case study: Mrs V

Mrs V is a resident of a nursing home and has been ambulant, social and apparently healthy for the past two years. The reason for her admission was social isolation, memory loss and a past history of falls with bilateral hip replacements prior to admission. Within the home, she was able to feed herself and attend to some hygiene needs, but required assistance with toileting and dressing. Her mobility was becoming an issue, as she appeared to be bumping into furniture and people, and on assessment it was discovered she was developing glaucoma. Over the period of a week, Mrs V seemed listless, more confused than usual, refused food and fluids and couldn't walk. Nursing staff took her temperature 37.5°C, pulse 90, respiration 24, blood pressure 100/50. Urinalysis revealed no ketones; protein was present and a specific gravity of 1030.

The conclusion was a urinary tract infection, and a culture and sensitivity specimen were dispatched to the laboratory. The results confirmed an infection and appropriate antibiotics were prescribed and administered. Extra fluids were offered but refused and cranberry tablets were administered. Four days later, Mrs V's confusion was worse and she appeared dehydrated and ill. Blood was sent for electrolytes, glucose and cell counts. Serum osmolality was 360 mOsm/L, white cell count elevated, sodium 155 mmol/L, potassium 5.5 mmol/L, blood glucose 17 mmol/L. The concluding diagnosis was untreated Type II diabetes with hyperglycaemic, hyperosmolar, non-ketotic syndrome. She required immediate hospitalisation and intravenous fluid replacement with dextrose/saline and insulin.

conclusion

There are several main observable features of fluid and/or electrolyte imbalance associated with the risk factors listed in this chapter. These are the common symptoms that nurses can assess and then begin to put into place necessary interventions to prevent the situation becoming worse. Routine observation of the physical appearance and reported behaviour or personality changes in older people are often the only methods of detecting the first signs of impending fluid and electrolyte imbalance. This is especially important for older people who have cognitive impairment and cannot convey symptoms of discomfort. A checklist of risk factors can be developed for assistance in assessing the potential for imbalances and a recognition of the need for preventive strategies to improve the wellbeing of older people is implementing best practice (see Appendix 9.1).

study questions

1   What are the major fluid compartments of concern in older people?
2   Why should oedema be treated seriously?
3   What are the types of oedema commonly observed in older people?
4   Why are older people prone to dehydration?
5   How can diabetes mellitus affect fluid and electrolyte balance?
6   Identify the risk factors for imbalance in older people.

references

Dargarville, R. (1995), *Diabetes Management Health Professional Symposium*, Diabetes Australia, Melbourne.

Groer, M. E. and Shekleton M. E. (1979), *Basic Pathophysiology: A Conceptual Approach*, C. V. Mosby, St Louis, Missouri.

Guyton, A. C. (1979), *Textbook of Medical Physiology*, 5th edn, W. B. Saunders Co, Philadelphia.

Hamilton, H. (ed.) (1982), 'Monitoring fluid and electrolytes precisely', *Nursing Skillbook Series*, Springhouse Corporation, Springhouse, Pennsylvania.

Holmes, H. N. (ed.) (1997), *Mastering Geriatric Care*, Springhouse Corporation, Springhouse, Pennsylvania.

Vander, A. J., Sherman, J. H. and Luciano, D. S. (1986), *Human Physiology: The Mechanisms of Body Function*, 4th edn, McGraw Hill, New York.

Vardaxis, N. J. (1994), *Pathology for the Health Sciences*, Macmillan Education, Melbourne.

Appendix 9.1: Assessment of alteration in fluid and electrolyte balance

Name: _____ Date: _____

Questions	Yes	Measure	No	Comments
1 Is there alteration in consciousness?		Pupil check		
2 Is there mental confusion (non-dementia)?		Cognitive check		
3 Is there obvious swelling of legs?		Pitting present		
4 Is there rapid pulse?		Check apex beat		
5 Are there breathing problems?		Lying or sitting		
6 Is there hypertension?		Check lying and standing		
7 Is there pain present?		Where		
8 Are there abnormal urine tests?		Protein, blood		
9 Are there known diagnoses such as diabetes mellitus, kidney disease etc?				
10 What medication is being taken that may alter the balance (eg, diuretics)?				
11 Is there a high temperature?				
12 Is there chronic infection?				
13 Is there repeated infection?				
14 Has there been vomiting?				
15 Has there been a rapid weight gain?		Daily weights		
16 Is there evidence of poor nutrition?		Weight and general appearance		
17 Are there muscle spasms or twitches?		Where		
18 Are there tremors (non-Parkinson's)?				
19 Is there obvious trauma (fractures)?				
20 Is there depression and non-eating?				
21 Has there been diarrhoea?		No. of stools		
22 Is there evidence of hyperventilation?				
23 Is there impaired swallowing?		TIAs, stroke		
24 Is there evidence of sun-burn?				
25 Should you do blood gases?				

From the answers to the above questions, you should be assisted to make a clinical decision as to how you could verify your conclusions and follow up with laboratory tests, further investigations, referral or observe further.

nutrition assessment and screening

Yvonne Coleman

chapter summary

Nutritional assessment is multi-factorial and nutritional management requires a multi-disciplinary approach. Nutritional assessment entails a combination of medical history, biochemical markers, drug–nutrient interactions, social history, anthropometric data and dietary assessment. This chapter offers a comprehensive guide to factors affecting the daily nutritional intake of older people and some assessment tools as examples for data collection.

learning objectives

After reading and reflecting on this chapter, you will be able to:

- create an awareness in health professionals of the importance of good nutritional status in older people
- create an awareness of the indirect effects of malnutrition
- create an awareness of the importance of screening for malnutrition
- provide some examples of screening tools that may be the basis of those used by an individual organisation
- provide some markers that may be used to assess the degree of malnutrition, and monitor the effect of interventions
- provide a tool for standardising stool descriptions
- create an awareness of some of the losses associated with enteral feeding.

introduction

The health status of older people is characterised by multimorbidity, chronic diseases, and physical, mental and social disabilities. More and longer hospital stays, slower recoveries from disease and higher risks of mortality influence the nutrition and nutritional status of older people (Volkert et al., 1992). Assessment of nutritional status in the elderly is important because acute and chronic diseases usually increase nutritional requirements. A mildly malnourished older person rapidly becomes acutely malnourished when their metabolic needs increase due to infection or tissue loss. This is generally overlooked in the chronically debilitated person (eg, with an oozing wound or a pressure area). Non-recognition of nutritional status often leads to complications that prolong wound healing or illness, and consequently increase medical care costs (Ham, 1994). Nutritional assessment entails a combination of medical history, biochemical markers, drug–nutrient interactions, social history, anthropometric data and dietary assessment.

medical history

Nutritional status at time of admission correlates with the risk of subsequent complications (Sullivan et al., 1990). The medical history can indicate both direct and indirect factors affecting nutritional status. Direct factors include diagnoses with a known nutritional component such as diabetes, coeliac disease, anaemia and constipation. Indirect factors, whereby nutritional status is either a contributing or an independent risk factor, include depression, dysphagia, dementia, fractures, falls, chest infections and pressure areas. Nutritional status influences morbidity and mortality outcomes, and is potentially correctable (Sullivan, Walls and Lipschitz, 1991).

swallowing difficulties

An impaired swallow reflex is indicated by a cough when swallowing and/or frequent chest infections. A speech pathology assessment is recommended. An individual can still maintain their nutritional status while requiring texture-modified foods and fluids. Loss of weight is a prime indicator that insufficient food is being provided to meet the nutritional needs of the individual, independently of the quantity provided on the plate. Texture-modified foods include soft, chopped, minced, vitamised, or pureed consistencies; and texture-modified fluids include nectar, honey, pouring cream or jelled fluids.

food intake

Nutritional status is dependent upon an adequate intake of foods and fluids. The provision of an appropriate diet is of no value unless eaten. Changes in taste, smell, sight, hearing and touch are unavoidable effects of ageing and these adversely affect food intake and limit the elderly person's ability to enjoy eating (Opheim and Wesselman, 1990), because:

- decreased numbers of taste buds and decreased taste acuity result in a loss of ability to detect sweet and salty, though not bitter and sour
- impaired vision affects the ability to distinguish foods
- decreased sense of smell makes it difficult to identify the aroma of foods and enjoy their flavour
- hearing impairment leads to reluctance to become involved in conversational situations such as in the (noisy) dining room
- poor dentition, ill-fitting dentures, and periodontal disease contribute to chewing problems and difficulty selecting appropriate foods
- weakened grasp makes it difficult to hold cups, glasses and utensils
- functional impairments such as uncoordinated hand and arm functions for eating, and gait disorders, interfere with access to food (Ham, 1994).

malnutrition

Malnutrition is an inability to maintain an acceptable weight due to the inappropriate intake, absorption or utilisation of food. It is very important that malnutrition in older people is not attributed to poor food intake alone, unless strong evidence exists for this. Underlying active medical problems and adverse drug reactions need to be addressed. Indicators of poor nutritional status (White et al., 1991) include:

- hypoalbuminaemia: albumin is less than 35 g/L
- low body weight: women less than 45 kg; men less than 50 kg
- change in functional status from 'independent' to 'dependent' in two of the following aids to daily living (ADLs): bathing, dressing, toileting, transferring, continence and/or feeding

- sustained inappropriate food intake: meal and snack frequency, quantity and quality of food choices, dietary modifications (both prescribed and self-imposed), alcohol abuse
- acute and chronic diseases including weight change, cognitive and/or emotional impairment such as dementia and depression, oral health problems, sensory impairment
- nutrition-related disorders including osteoporosis, folate deficiency, or vitamin B12 deficiency
- chronic medication use including prescribed and/or self-administered medication, polypharmacy, nutritional supplements
- pressure areas: there is high risk when serum albumin is less than 33 g/L and total lymphocyte count is less than 1400 nm (Pinchcofsky-Devin and Kaminski, 1986).
- falls: malnutrition may decrease muscle mass with resultant weakness and gait abnormalities; it may also affect protective mechanisms, such as reaction time, movement coordination, and muscle strength; or indicate deficiencies in nutrients such as vitamin B12 (loss of position sense) and potassium (muscle weakness) (Vellas et al., 1991)

Consequences of malnutrition include increased risk of infection; respiratory problems; skin breakdown and ulceration; delayed or poor wound healing; prolonged post-operative complications; reduced muscle strength; poor mobility; fractured hip; cardiac difficulties such as altered electrocardiogram; apathy, irritability, memory loss, confusion; loss of functional capacity; increased length of hospital stay; and increased mortality; all of which add to increased nursing time and medical costs. Malnutrition is resolving when there is improving appetite and a slow and steady weight gain trend, resolving pressure areas, and improving nutritional biochemical markers.

hydration

Many older people mistakenly believe that a reduction in fluid intake will reduce their incontinence. Thirst sensitivity decreases with age, and an inadequate fluid intake contributes to incontinence, constipation, confusion, and loss of appetite. An adequate fluid intake can be calculated as 30 mL/kg body weight per day with a minimum requirement of 1500 mL/day (Chernoff, 1994) or can be counted as eight to ten cups per day.

constipation

Constipation is a subjective interpretation of bowel motions and includes infrequent defecation, excessive strain during defecation, small or hard stools, or a sense of incomplete evacuation (Wald, 1993). Poor hydration results in water being absorbed from the large intestine in an attempt to maintain fluid levels. This produces hard, dry faeces that may irritate the mucosa of the rectum and colon, causing excess mucous production. The mucous may dissolve some faeces, which then passes through as loose stool and causes soiling, which may be misinterpreted as faecal incontinence. Consequently, constipation may present as faecal incontinence (Hunt, 1993).

Unless the person is fluid restricted for medical reasons, then a fluid intake of eight to ten cups of non-alcoholic fluid per day is recommended. A diet of mainly refined foods with few fruits and vegetables, breads and cereals, predisposes to constipation because there is insufficient bulk to stimulate peristaltic action. The recommended intake of fibre is 25–40 g per day. Thirty grams of fibre intake per day can be achieved with three fruit serves, plus four to five vegetable serves, plus six serves of wholemeal breads and cereals. Constipation due to dietary factors is preventable. An adequate fluid intake and a high fibre diet are recommended.

bowels

A rectal examination may indicate diarrhoea, constipation, faecal impaction, or even occult or frank bleeding (Chandra et al., 1991). A standardised descriptive format is necessary to describe stool frequency and consistency, especially when assessing the effectiveness of treatment. Beverley and Travis (1992) devised the following:

1 Watery.
2 Liquid, creamy.
3 Very loose, mushy semi-liquid.
4 Loose, soft.
5 Formed with some liquid.
6 Soft, formed.
7 Normal, formed.
8 Hard.
9 Hard, dry.

immune system

Well-nourished people catch fewer infections less often and with less severity than malnourished people. All infections reduce nutrient intakes, increase nutrient losses, and increase the requirements for energy and protein. A single acute episode of infection does not usually cause much harm; however, the pattern of chronic infection, or frequent infections without time for full recovery in between, promotes nutrient losses and results in malnutrition. It is a universal practice to not serve solid foods to individuals with fever, diarrhoea or other symptoms of infection. The purposeful withholding of food plus infection-induced anorexia, contribute to the development of malnutrition.

Acute and/or chronic infections worsen any past dietary deficiencies. Correction of these deficiencies, especially while the infection persists, is very difficult by diet alone. The diet during the convalescent period influences whether a full recovery is effected before another infection occurs. Many people, however, find it difficult to eat a sufficient quantity to replenish body stores. When there are chronic or frequent infections, it becomes difficult to reverse the consequent malnutrition, which in turn lowers one's resistance to more infections.

diabetes

Nutritional management of people with diabetes is important for maintaining good control and reducing the risk of complications. Low blood sugar levels may be due to medications or to an inappropriate diet; and high blood sugar levels may be due to infection, medications, or inappropriate diet. Basic guidelines for good diabetes control are:

- regular meals at regular times
- a starchy food at each meal (bread, rice, pasta, potatoes, porridge, etc)
- between-meal snacks if there is more than four hours between meals
- supper if people have disturbed sleep, especially if they are taking medications for diabetes.

Currently there is controversy internationally regarding diabetes education formats. The preferred option in Australia is based on the glycaemic index, which indicates rates of absorption of the different sugars in foods; in the United States it is based on the monitoring of total carbohydrate intake such as an exchange system; while some European countries have developed a liberalised approach.

artificial nutritional support

Artificial nutritional support is introduced as a medical treatment and excludes the sensory, social and cultural pleasures and traditions associated with eating. Introduction of enteral or parenteral feeding necessitates a grieving response—grieving the loss of eating. This concept is rarely recognised by health professionals and the person may be labelled as 'depressed'. Unique losses associated with artificial feeding, include:

- Altered body image due to placement of the feeding tube: individuals may feel self-conscious about their appearance, which hinders their ability to maintain social normality. While G-tubes can be hidden beneath clothing, naso-gastric tubes are blatantly obvious and may result in social isolation.
- Altered family dynamics: the individual may be unable to perform the necessary connection procedures which then results in loss of independence; family members may feel uncomfortable cooking and eating foods that the enterally-fed person is unable to eat (Srp et al., 1989); food is not consumed at regular mealtimes and may be given continuously throughout the 24-hour day, or at times of the day other than the commonly recognised mealtimes (eg, even while asleep) (Bayer, Bauers and Kapp, 1983).
- Sensory deprivation: especially taste, texture, colour, chewing and swallowing food; drinking liquids; unsatisfied appetite for certain foods (eg, chocolate); gut stimulation due to chewing, satiety (Padilla and Grant 1985).

The two main forms of artificial nutritional support are enteral feeding and parenteral feeding.

enteral feeding

Enteral feeding is initiated when a person has a functional gastro-intestinal tract and is not eating adequately to maintain weight. The type of enteral feeding is dependent upon both individual requirements and the anticipated length of time of enteral feeding. The three types of enteral feeding are:

- Naso-gastric: tube insertion via the nose into the stomach. This is recommended for short-term use only (ie, two to three weeks).
- Gastrostomy: typically called a G-tube. The tube is inserted directly into the stomach, usually by the percutaneous endoscopic gastro-

stomy (PEG) procedure. Starter tubes establish the tract, and are patent for about six months. Replacement tubes are used once the tract has been established and are typically held in position with a balloon; these are patent for about 12–24 months. Gastrostomy is recommended for long-term use (ie, if required for a longer period of time than two to three weeks).

- Jejunostomy: tube insertion through a gastrostomy tract to the jejunum. These are managed similarly to gastrostomies. They are currently not common.

Feeding regimens can be bolus, intermittent or continuous:

- Bolus feeding is the provision of a small amount of formula, typically approximately 300 mL, that is either gravity fed or syringed into the tube in a short period of time, usually five to six times per day. There may be problems with tolerance and increased risk of chest infections.
- Intermittent feeding is the provision of a greater volume of formula over a longer period of time, typically three times per day, and usually regulated by an enteral feeding pump. There are fewer problems with intolerance and chest infections with this regimen. This method of feeding promotes the concept of feeding to approximate meal times, and may facilitate improved diabetes control.
- Continuous feeding is the provision of a defined amount of formula over 20–24 hours, and is usually regulated by an enteral feeding pump. There are fewer problems with intolerance with this method, but there is an increased risk of chest infections due to lying flat while feeding at night.

Standard enteral formulas provide 1 kCal/mL. Specialised formulas may provide fibre, or increased energy density (eg, 2 kCal/mL). The use of infant formula or vitamised food is *not* advised. An excellent resource organisation for health professionals is the Gastrostomy Information and Support Society, PO Box 381, St Kilda, Victoria 3182, Phone: 03 9537 2611.

parenteral feeding

Parenteral feeding is initiated when a person has a dysfunctional gastro-intestinal tract and is not eating adequately to maintain weight.

Although the ability to eat is fundamental to our survival, the impact of its loss as a unique loss is rarely recognised.

drug–nutrient interactions

Drugs can affect nutritional status by altering the intake, absorption, metabolism and excretion of nutrients, and nutritional status can affect the absorption, distribution, metabolism, and excretion of drugs.

effects of drugs on nutritional status

Mechanisms by which drugs can affect nutritional status include:

- Altered food intake—suppression or stimulation of appetite:
  - drugs associated with increased appetite include antipsychotic agents and some antihistamines such as cyproheptadine
  - decreased appetite may be due to side effects such as diarrhoea, constipation, anorexia, nausea, vomiting, and altered taste perception. Who wants to eat with any of these side effects, especially if they are present with any degree of severity?
- Interference with nutrient absorption—primarily by malabsorption. The drug binds with the nutrient and prevents absorption of drug, nutrient or both. Examples include thyroxine and iron, tetracyclines, and calcium, magnesium, iron and zinc (Coleman, 1998).
- Alteration in nutrient metabolism: some drugs increase nutrient metabolism and consequently increase nutrient requirements. An example is phenytoin and vitamins D, K, and folate.
- Increased nutrient excretion: drugs that have this effect include aspirin (which affects vitamin D, calcium, vitamin B12, iron, potassium, vitamins K and C, folate and glucose), potassium (which affects vitamin B12), and the thiazide diuretics (which affect potassium, magnesium, zinc, sodium and calcium) (Coleman, 1998).

effects of nutritional mechanisms on drug availability

Some of the nutritional mechanisms that can affect drug availability are as follows:

- Malnutrition: this usually results in reduced plasma proteins, which are the primary transporters for drugs such as frusemide, digoxin, warfarin and tetracyclines (Caswell et al., 1998). For example, hypoalbuminaemia may exacerbate a high INR (International Normalised Ratio) result for people on warfarin.

- Mixing of drugs in foods or drinks may result in the formation of unpalatable and insoluble precipitates (Pronsky, 1995). For example, adding drugs to an enteral formula can cause the drugs to precipitate and thus reduce their effectiveness, and may also cause a blocked tube.
- Food–drug interactions can have a variety of undesirable effects on drug action (Pronsky, 1995). For example, caffeine negates the effects of sedatives.
- Nutrient–drug interactions may affect drug utilisation. For example, if iron supplements are given simultaneously with levodopa, then there is possible chelation of drug and supplement and a result of reduced antiparkinson effect.
- Nutritional adverse reactions have unpleasant side effects such as gastrointestinal disturbances, appetite changes, a dry or sore mouth, or altered taste perceptions. People may decide to gain relief by reducing or eliminating certain foods from the diet, not eating, using over-the-counter drugs, or may discontinue using the drug (Pronsky, 1995).

social history

Food and eating have social, psychological and physiological roles (Bayer, Bauers and Kapp, 1983). Emotional factors influence our attitudes to, and choices of food. Social history information can include domestic arrangements. For example, Does the person live alone? Who does the cooking? Can they cook? Do they receive Meals on Wheels, and (more importantly) do they eat the Meals on Wheels? How long have they been cooking for themselves? Are there food restrictions that they cater to (eg, avoiding 'acid' foods because of arthritis)? Do they use multivitamins? Do they skip meals? Is there a variety in their meals (ie, are there choices from all of the five food groups)? How are their groceries supplied? Is there a caregiver available with the time to assist feeding? Can they afford to buy food?

anthropometric data

Anthropometric measurements indicate body composition. Although there are several measures, the most common are weight and height measurements. Body weight indicates the total composition of protein, fat, water and bone mass, but does not indicate changes in these four compartments. There is a tendency to increase fat deposition with age, along with a reduction in muscle protein. Conditions such as oedema, ascites or tumour growth may mask body composition changes (Gibson, 1993). Weights are affected by time of day, meal intake, and bowel and bladder content.

Weight loss correlates with morbidity and mortality (Lipkin and Bell, 1993). The optimal cut-off point for defining clinically important weight loss is in the 4–5 per cent range (ie, about 2–3 kg in a person who weighs 50–60 kg). A detailed weight history is capable of predicting hospital-based morbidity with an acceptable level of sensitivity, and costs nothing (Lipkin and Bell, 1993). Routine recording of weights at the time of admission and discharge, and serially (eg, weekly during the length of stay) is strongly recommended.

Age-related shrinking of the spinal column may compromise height measurements. Stature may be calculated by measuring the 'wingspan' of individuals (ie, finger-tip to finger-tip). This measurement gives a very good approximation of stature with minimal difficulty, and is suitable for people who have kyphosis or are amputees.

dietary assessment

Dietary assessment methods usually consist of food intake recalls, or food records designed to measure the quantity of foods consumed over a period of time. The 24-hour recall provides information on the person's food intake during the previous 24 hours. Its success depends on the individual's memory, their ability to convey accurate estimates of portion sizes consumed (Gibson, 1993) and the customariness of that day's food intake.

The three-day food record is usually based on the food intake of two week days and one weekend day, to take into account the potential differences in food consumption patterns. Participants may, however, change their usual eating pattern to simplify the process (Gibson, 1993). This method is primarily used in research when accuracy is important. Nutrient intakes can be calculated from the food composition values available in food composition tables or nutrient databases.

nutrition screening tools

Nutrition screening is a cost-effective method for assessing the degree of nutritional risk. There are currently three simple, effective screening tools available in Australia: nutritional risk screening and monitoring, nutrition risk screening for community rehabilitation centre clients, and the Australian Nutrition Screening Initiative.

nutritional risk screening and monitoring

This method was developed by Dr Bev Woods in conjunction with the Victorian Home and Community Care Program (1998). See Appendix 10.1 for an outline of this nutritional risk screening and monitoring tool.

Since 1998, a Victorian project, *Identifying and Assisting People who are Nutritionally at Risk* (Wood, 1998), has successfully developed a number of resources, all to support the identification of, and provision of assistance to, home-based frail, elderly people who are nutritionally at risk. If a vulnerable person can be prevented from risk of nutritional health problems or if a condition of nutritional risk can be reversed or ameliorated, premature frailty and/or ill health can be avoided, as well as premature admission to an institution. Food and nutrition problems can be solved by a general health professional providing effective support to the person, or by a specialist in food and nutrition issues who can provide more expert assistance. This simple and quick method of nutritional risk screening for home-based clients (Wood, Stewart and Race, 1998) can be used in association with any assessment form or process. Further nutritional risk screening is embedded in the general assessment conducted with the client, and will probably reveal the reasons why the client is at nutritional risk.

Identifying and Planning Assistance to Home Based Adults who are Nutritionally at Risk. A Resource Manual (Wood, Stewart and Race, 1998) has been designed to demonstrate and advocate for the introduction of nutritional risk screening to the assessment process for all frail, elderly clients who require community services to remain in their own homes. This manual explains the basis of nutritional risk screening and the tool that has been developed. It also gives many practical suggestions about solving client problems, and information on where further assistance may be sought.

In developing these materials, the basic tenet of the Nutrition Screening Initiative (1992) has been used; that is, 'Nutrition screening and intervention are best accomplished by an interdisciplinary team . . . [that] uses existing programs and fosters collaboration amongst professionals' (ibid., p. 4).

nutrition risk screening for community rehabilitation centre clients

This method was developed by Debbie Wynd, chief dietitian at the Barton Health Grace McKellar Centre, Geelong, Victoria. See Appendix 10.2 for an outline of this nutrition risk screening tool.

the Australian nutrition screening initiative

This was developed by the Royal Australian College of General Practitioners, Council of the Ageing, Dietitians Association of Australia and Self Care Pharmacy (a joint program of the Pharmaceutical Society and Pharmacy Guild of Australia). See Appendix 10.3 for an outline of this initiative.

case history: Mrs R

Mrs R is an 83-year-old woman, who has been admitted to an interim extended care ward for evaluation of functional status.

- Her medical history includes two AMIs, cancer of cervix, COAD, frequent falls, frailty, hypertension, Parkinson's disease, peptic ulcer, cholecystectomy. Her social history includes living alone in her own home.
- Her biochemistry on admission was as follows: sodium 133 mmol/L, potassium 4.0 mmol/L, urea 8.4 mmol/L, creatinine 0.09 mmol/L, haemoglobin 12.2 g/L, lymphocytes 1.4 nL, albumin 31 g/L, total proteins 60 g/L.
- Her medications on admission (and their effects) are presented in Table 10.1.
- Her anthropometric data on admission: Weight not done, Height/wingspan not done.

initial nutritional assessment

Alcohol and liquorice both contra-indicated because of interactions with specific drugs. Medications may be affecting appetite and food intake, and have the potential to cause dry mouth and dysphagia. Visceral proteins (albumin and lymphocytes) indicate a high risk of pressure area formation. Both falls and frailty are independent risk factors for poor nutritional status. Cancer of the cervix, COAD and Parkinson's disease each increase nutrient requirements, and thus a high energy and nutri-

Table 10.1: *Medications on admission*

Drug	Nutrients affected	Nausea/ vomiting	Constipation/ diarrhoea	Weight loss/gain	Appetite
Ranitidine	B12, B1, iron	Yes	Yes		
Sinemet	B6, C, folate	Yes	Yes	Yes	Decreases
Oxazepam		Nausea	Constipation	Gain	Increases
Aspirin	D, calcium, potassium, iron, C, folate, vit K	Yes			Decreases
Ferrogradumet					
Salt tabs					
Panadeine forte			Constipation		Decreases
Zoloft		Yes	Yes	Yes	Decreases
Tritace		Yes	Yes		Decreases
Fosamax	Calcium	Yes	Yes		
Coloxyl + senna	Potassium, calcium, all vitamins	Yes	Diarrhoea, steatorrhoea	Decreases	

(Drug information compiled from Coleman, 1998)

ent-dense diet is required. Reports loss of weight of about one stone (6–7 kg) in the previous six months. Dislikes milky drinks; therefore, fruit juice based nutritional products are the preferred option for nutritional supplementation. Slight hyponatraemia may be associated with diabetes. Proposed discharge destination indeterminate.

initial nutritional plan

• To have nutritional product three times per day; at morning tea, afternoon tea and supper. Between-meal nutritional supplements allow gastric emptying prior to the next meal and therefore there is less interference with appetite for meals.

Altered taste	Dysphagia	Dry mouth	Thirst	Drooling	Blood sugar levels
	Yes	Yes			↑↓
		Yes			
					↑↓
		Yes			
Yes	Yes	Yes	Yes		
Yes	Yes	Yes			↑↓
Yes	Yes				
Yes					

- Weekly weighs to monitor adequacy of oral intake. Weight gain is desirable.
- Monitor biochemistry in three weeks to ensure nutritional markers are within the acceptable range.
- Check for diabetes.

during the course of her admission

- A slow weight gain trend was recorded.
- Improved response to physiotherapy and occupational therapy inputs.

- Fasting BSLs within the acceptable range; therefore, hyponatraemia must have an alternative cause.
- Hyponatraemia resolving, and salt tablets ceased.
- Complaints of dry mouth noted and some medications ceased.

at time of discharge

- Weight gain of at least 3 kg during admission.
- Discharged home.
- Biochemical nutritional markers within the acceptable range (low albumin status and/or loss of weight during admission are good predictors of non-elective readmission to an acute care institution).
- Nutritional support products ceased and still gaining weight (further weight gain of approximately 3–4 kg is desirable; appetite usually adjusts at end of convalescence).

summary

- Malnutrition was resolved as indicated by the nutritional biochemical markers, and improved response to physiotherapy and occupational therapy inputs.
- Discharged home, and without supports; the best outcome that could be achieved.
- Poor nutritional status contributed to the admission; appropriate diet therapy input contributed significantly to a good outcome.
- Non-recognition of poor nutritional status, and resolution of the problems, would have resulted in this woman being discharged to a nursing home unnecessarily.

conclusion

Nutritional assessment is multi-factorial, and nutritional management requires a multi-disciplinary approach. Underlying medical problems and adverse drug reactions must be identified and managed. Malnutrition in older people is a major health problem and has very negative health outcome implications. Poor nutritional status must not be blamed on poor nutritional intake unless there is very good evidence for this. Ongoing education for health professionals regarding malnutrition in older people needs to be promoted. Screening for nutritional status should become a routine part of the medical and health assessments of older people (Lipski, 1995).

abbreviations

AMI	acute myocardial infarction
BSL	blood sugar level
COAD	chronic obstructive airways disease
CRC	community rehabilitation centre
GISS	Gastrostomy Information and Support Society
IWR	ideal weight for range
PEG	percutaneous endoscopic gastrostomy

references

Bayer, L. M., Bauers, C. M. and Kapp, S. R. (1983), 'Psychosocial aspects of nutritional support', *Nursing Clinics of North America*, 18(1), pp. 119–28.

Beverley, L. and Travis, I. (1992), 'Constipation: Proposed natural laxative mixtures', *Journal of Gerontological Nursing*, 10, pp. 5–12.

Caswell, A., Badewitz-Dodd, L. H., Littlemore, L., Gold, R. and Middlin, P. (eds) (1998), *1998 MIMS Annual. Australian Edition*, MediMedia Australia Pty Ltd, Sydney.

Chandra, R. K., Imbach, A., Moore, C., Skelton, D. and Woolcott, D. (1991), 'Nutrition of the elderly', *Canadian Medical Association Journal*, 145(11), pp. 1475–87.

Chernoff, R. (1994), 'Meeting the nutritional needs of the elderly in the institutional setting', *Nutrition Reviews*, 52(4), pp. 132–6.

Coleman, Y. (1998), *Drug–Nutrient Interactions: The Manual*, Nutrition Consultants Australia, Melbourne.

Gibson, R. A. (1993), *Nutritional Assessment: A Laboratory Manual*, Oxford University Press, New York.

Ham, R. J. (1994), 'The signs and symptoms of poor nutritional status', *Primary Care*, 21(1), pp. 33–54.

Hunt, S. (1993), *Promoting Continence in the Nursing Home*, Continence Foundation of Australia, Sydney.

Lipkin, E. W. and Bell, S. (1993), 'Assessment of nutritional status', *Clinics in Laboratory Medicine*, 13(2), pp. 329–52.

Lipski, P. S. (1995), 'The consequences of undernutrition in the elderly', *Proceedings of the Nutrition Society of Australia*, 19, pp. 146–51.

Nutrition Screening Initiative (1992), *The Nutritional Intervention Manual for Professionals Caring For Older Americans*, Vol. Definitions, Nutrition Screening Initiative, Washington DC.

Opheim, C. and Wesselman, J. (1990), 'Optimal dietary prescribing in the nursing home', *Geriatrics*, 45(7), pp. 66–71.

Padilla, G. V. and Grant, M. M. (1985), 'Psychosocial aspects of artificial feeding', *Cancer*, 55(1), pp. 301–4.

Pinchcofsky-Devin, G. D. and Kaminski, M. (1986): Correlation of pressure sores and nutritional status, *Journal of the American Geriatrics Society* 34: 435–440.

Pronsky, Z. M. (1995): *Food Medication Interactions*. 9th Ed. Food-Medication Interactions, Pottstown.

Srp, F., Steiger, E., Gulledge, A. D., Matarese, L. E., Paysinger, J., Roncagli, T., Stebbins, J. and Sullivan, M. (1989), 'Psychosocial issues of nutritional support: A multidisciplinary interpretation', *Nursing Clinics of North America*, 24(2), pp. 447–59.

Sullivan, D. H., Patch, G. A., Walls, R. C. and Lipschitz, D. A. (1990), 'Impact of nutrition status on morbidity and mortality in a select population of geriatric rehabilitation patients', *American Journal of Clinical Nutrition*, 51, pp. 749–58.

Sullivan, D. H., Walls, R. C. and Lipschitz, D. A. (1991), 'Protein–energy undernutrition and the risk of mortality within 1 year of hospital discharge in a select population of geriatric rehabilitation patients', *American Journal of Clinical Nutrition*, 53, pp. 599–605.

Vellas, B., Baumgartner, R. N., Wayne, S. J., Conceicao, J., Lafont, C., Albarede, J-L. and Garry, P. J. (1991), 'Relationship between malnutrition and falls in the elderly', *Nutrition*, 8 (2), pp. 105–8.

Volkert, D., Kruse, W., Oster, P. and Schlierf, G. (1992), 'Malnutrition in geriatric patients: Diagnostic and prognostic significance of nutritional parameters', *Annals of Nutrition and Metabolism*, 36, pp. 97–112.

Wald, A. (1993), 'Constipation in elderly patients: Pathogenesis and management', *Drugs and Aging*, 3(3), pp. 220–31.

White, J. V., Ham, R. J., Lipschitz, D. A., Dwyers, J. T. and Wellman, N. S. (1991), 'Consensus of the nutrition screening initiative: Risk factors and indicators of poor nutritional status in older Americans', *Journal of the American Dietitians Association*, 91(7), pp. 783–7.

Wood, B. (ed.) (1998), *Identifying and Assisting People who are Nutritionally at Risk: Third Report*, Dietitians Association of Australia (Victorian Branch), Melbourne.

Wood, B., Stewart, A. and Race, S. (eds) (1998), *Identifying and Planning Assistance to Home Based Adults who are Nutritionally at Risk. A Resource Manual*, Dietitians Association of Australia (Victorian Branch), Melbourne.

Appendix 10.1: Nutritional risk screening and monitoring

Victorian Home and Community Care Program (1998)	
NUTRITIONAL RISK SCREENING AND MONITORING	
Client:	**Date:**
Π Obvious underweight/frailty Π Unintentional weight loss	
Π Reduced appetite or food and fluid intake	
Π Mouth or teeth or swallowing problem	
Π Follows a special diet	
Π Unable to shop for food Π Unable to prepare food	
Π Unable to feed self	
Π Obvious overweight affecting life quality Π Unintentional weight gain	
Signature:	**Position:**

- **Yes** to one or more questions means that nutritional risk exists.
- Nutritional risk increases when the person is affected by an increasing number of general needs assessment factors.
- In particular, deterioration in health and loss of independence can result from undernutrition and perhaps malnutrition.
- Try **two** weeks of simple intervention strategies (less time if severe weight loss). If no response, refer to a specialist.
- Monitoring at monthly intervals (or more frequently) is then recommended by one of the team members, to ensure that the most effective intervention has been implemented.

Appendix 10.2: Nutrition risk screening for community rehabilitation centre clients tool

instructions

Complete as part of the routine nursing assessment process for all new clients attending CRC. If 'yes' is the answer, then tick the box. One or more ticks indicates nutritional risk, and the more ticks then the greater the risk.

If any of these first four questions are ticked, then refer to the dietitian.

Obvious underweight/frailty (see chart below: if ≥5 kg under ideal weight for range, then refer to dietitian)
Obvious overweight affecting life quality (see chart: if ≥5 kg over IWR, then refer to dietitian)
Unintentional weight loss (if > ~2 kg over four weeks, then refer to dietitian)
Follows a special diet and has not had a review by a dietitian within the past 12 months/requests review

If any of the next four questions are ticked, then determine the degree of the problem and address accordingly (eg, provide advice, refer to appropriate health professional or community service, etc). If two or more boxes are ticked, then refer to dietitian.

Follows a special diet and has had a review by a dietitian within the past 12 months
Reduced appetite or food/fluid intake
Mouth, teeth or swallowing problem
Unable to shop, prepare food or feed self adequately

Appendix 10.2: (continued)

This chart shows the best weight range for people over 65 years.

Height	Ideal weight range
147 cm	57.7 kg–58.6 kg
150 cm	49.5 kg–60.8 kg
152 cm	51.1 kg–62.7 kg
155 cm	52.8 kg–64.7 kg
158 cm	54.6 kg–67.0 kg
160 cm	56.3 kg–69.1 kg
163 cm	58.2 kg–71.4 kg
165 cm	59.9 kg–73.5 kg
168 cm	61.8 kg–75.8 kg
170 cm	63.6 kg–78.0 kg
173 cm	65.6 kg–81.9 kg
175 cm	67.4 kg–82.7 kg
178 cm	69.6 kg–85.4 kg
180 cm	71.3 kg–87.5 kg
183 cm	73.5 kg–90.2 kg

Appendix 10.3: Australian nutrition screening initiative

The warning signs of poor nutritional health in the older person are often overlooked. Use this checklist to find out if you or someone you know is at nutritional risk. Read the statements below. Circle the number in the column that applies to you. Total your nutritional score.

	Yes	No
I have an illness or condition that made me change the kind and/or amount of food I eat.	2	0
I eat at least three meals per day.	0	3
I eat fruit or vegetables most days.	0	2
I eat dairy products most days.	0	2
I have three or more glasses of beer, wine or spirits almost every day.	3	0
I have six to eight cups of fluids (eg, water, juice, tea or coffee) most days.	0	1
I have teeth, mouth or swallowing problems that make it hard for me to eat.	4	0
I always have enough money to buy food.	0	3
I eat alone most of the time.	2	0
I take three or more different prescribed or over-the-counter medicines every day.	3	0
Without wanting to, I have lost or gained 5 kg in the last six months.	2	0
I am always able to shop, cook and/or feed myself.	0	2
Total		

Add up all the numbers you have circled. If your nutritional score is . . .

0–3   **Good!** Recheck your nutritional score in six months.

4–5   **You are at moderate nutritional risk**. See what can be done to improve your eating habits and lifestyle. Your Council on Ageing or health care professionals can help. Recheck your nutritional score in three months.

6 or more   **You are at high nutritional risk.** Bring this checklist the next time you see your doctor, dietitian or other qualified health or social service professional. Talk with them about any problems you may have. Ask for help to improve your nutritional health.

chapter 11

assessment of palliation

Jenny Abbey

chapter summary

This chapter outlines the issues surrounding palliative care for older people, especially those in residential care settings. The concept of quality of life is discussed and the necessity for a team approach in providing palliation for older people at the end stage of life.

objectives

After reading and reflecting on this chapter, you will be able to:

- identify the need for palliation in residential care settings
- discuss the relevance of team work in palliative care
- analyse the clinical interventions that may be required to fulfil quality palliative care.

introduction

Nurses perceive palliative care in aged care settings in a variety of ways. The views range from 'we do it all the time here', where all care is considered palliative, to 'we can't do that here'. The latter comment is usually followed by an explanation of the philosophy of the facility or the beliefs of the patients' families which impede discussion or implementation of anything but a cure-oriented and keep-alive-at-all-costs approach.

This situation will need to be clarified as palliative care becomes more mainstream due to the fact that it is now assessable for both monetary compensation and for accreditation standards. Also, in future, nurses will be expected to be able to respond to care demands driven by quality of life measures as consumers absorb messages from the increasing media coverage about death issues. O'Boyle and Waldron (1997, p. 18) explain the new wave of thinking that is occurring:

> The assessment of patients' quality of life is assuming increasing importance in medicine and health care. Illnesses, diseases and their treatments can have significant impacts on such areas of functioning as mobility, mood, life satisfaction, sexuality, cognition, and ability to fulfil occupational, social and family roles. The emerging quality of life construct may be viewed as a paradigm shift in outcome measurement since it shifts the focus of attention from symptoms to functioning. This holistic approach more clearly establishes the patient as the centre of attention and subsumes many of the traditional measures of outcome. Quality of life assessment is particularly relevant to patients with progressive conditions, particularly in the later phases of the disease.

This change to a different contextual framework for assessment *will* take place, and as it does, a move towards a universally accepted frame of reference for care and documentation of palliative care, for both the acutely and chronically ill elderly will be imperative.

The concept of palliative care for someone with cancer can be introduced into conversation and discussed reasonably easily as the patient and their family ask questions about the progress of the disease and an estimate of how long it will take to die. In the case of an older person, the first step in the palliative care process, raising the subject, is much more difficult. Euphemisms about seeking help to die are often employed by the young and middle-aged. 'Shoot me if I get like that' or 'just push me off my perch' are commonplace if the subject of dementia or other incurable debilitating diseases of old age are discussed. Certainly, this is often the reaction on someone's first visit to an aged care facility. As people get older, this certainty about wanting to be helped to die often becomes less intense. However, the conviction of not wanting to suffer unbearably is almost universal and usually does not change as death approaches. This is the difference between palliative care and euthanasia. Palliative care is about caring but not curing. The complex arguments within the euthanasia debate about double-effect, the slippery slope, letting die versus killing, starving versus withdrawing food and fluid and so on are set out in many other publications (Charlesworth, 1993; Kuhse, 1994; Singer, 1994; Tonti-Filippini, 1994; Royal College of Nursing, Australia, 1995) and do not have a place here. This chapter is concerned with how to implement an agreed palliative care program for older people outside a hospice setting.

case conferences, documentation and making a choice

The timing of the introduction of palliative care, especially for the elderly with chronic, slowly developing conditions is an area where very little research has been undertaken. It has been found that health professionals emphasise the more traditional concept of palliative care (eg, relief from pain) as people get obviously close to death (Lowden, 1998). But palliative care for the elderly has to be more than that. Before a palliative care service can be introduced, the following preliminary steps need to be in place:

- a written philosophy of the organisation, reflecting support for individual choice of care, including palliative care
- an education program that assists staff to clarify their values and attitudes, as well as learning clinical aspects of palliative care
- established connections with palliative care specialists, both medical and nursing
- a well established and managed system of case conferences where decisions are made by and with all concerned parties and then clearly documented
- multi-disciplinary care plans, where the patient's wishes and doctors', therapists' and nurses' actions and their care of a patient are documented in the patient's progress notes

- an established palliative care protocol, care map or clinical pathway that integrates interventions as well as measurement of outcomes.

Good communication between nurses and patients is a central aspect of palliative care. Research has found that an extensive communication skills program that allows nurses to explore attitudes, raise self-awareness and develop knowledge and skills appears to be effective (MacMahon and Thomas, 1998). Since it is unlikely that this kind of time-consuming education will be possible for all nurses working with older clients, the concept of an experienced palliative care nurse, who will take the major role in organising and running case conferences and communicating about palliative care interventions and outcomes to both client and family and friends, is probably the most realistic and effective way of managing. It may seem an impossible dream for every organisation to have access to, or to employ, a palliative care nurse specialist, but this was also the case for nurses who specialised in incontinence a decade ago.

What follows is a real case study, where staff of an aged care facility were assisted by the intervention of a palliative care nurse consultant. As you read this, it would be useful to work out how the staff could have coped alone if the steps above had been implemented.

case study: palliative care assessment in the aged care setting

background

Max has been a resident of a metropolitan aged care facility for the last six years. He is 78 years old and has been widowed eight years. His only daughter works part-time and visits at least three times per week. He is a well-liked and 'treasured' resident of the hostel, according to staff.

previous medical history

- Long-term peripheral vascular disease, now with ischaemic pain with any exertion.
- Multiple previous arterial leg ulcers and amputation of toes of right foot, which has failed to heal completely.
- Hypertension.
- Hypercholestraemia.
- Osteoarthritis of hips and knees.

- Lumbar sympathectomy nine years ago.
- Heavy smoker of 50 years.

nursing history

Max's understanding and ability to reason are intact and he has always been keen to have a lot of control over his day-to-day activities. He was able to sit out in a chair and shower sitting until three months ago. Now he spends his time in bed and needs full care from the nursing staff. He has a poor appetite and drinks only when prompted, although he enjoys a small glass of beer in the evening.

On the assessment document completed previously, Max's legs were described as being pale, cool, absent pulse on right foot and very weak on left foot. Moderate pain was reported in both legs (right less so than left) when elevated or with any extended exertion. Pain scores were not documented. A necrotic wound was present on the right foot where the amputation had failed to heal. This was assessed as needing twice-daily dressings with the aim of removing the dead tissue and eventual healing.

current issues

Max has had extreme pain in both legs with any exertion and moderate pain at rest. Slowly escalating doses of morphine (initially 10 mg slow-release morphine twice daily, now 100 mg) are now not providing adequate analgesia, but associated nausea is worsening. Max says he is scared that he will develop a tolerance to the morphine such that he will need ever-increasing doses to maintain his comfort, eventually getting to the stage where it doesn't work at all. This is a common, but unfounded, fear. His right foot wound has become larger due to increased generalised body breakdown and is increasingly painful when dressed. The right lower leg is now cold and popliteal pulse is absent. The vascular surgeon strongly suggested an above-knee amputation as all other attempts to heal the wound have failed.

While he was in hospital, Max had met a number of people who were having amputations and this led him to say that he would rather die than let this happen to him. He has asked an RN on a number of occasions to 'put me out of my misery' and has said, 'They shoot animals don't they?'. He says he has made the decision to cease all food, fluids other than water (and his beer!) and medications (except analgesia) as this is just 'prolonging my suffering'. His daughter is very upset to hear this but tearfully says she understands his motives. Most nurses voice similar feelings and express their frustration at seeing Max suffering.

Max's general practitioner has ceased regular reviews, now visiting only when called by the hostel staff. The staff feel the GP is having trouble accepting Max's decision and does not want to be involved. As a clinical nurse specialist involved in providing palliative care consultation, support and education to aged care facilities, I was asked by the staff to become involved with Max's care to support him, his daughter and the nursing staff.

interventions

I discussed with Max his wishes to withdraw from all treatment except analgesia. He reiterated to me his wishes and was clear about the implications of this. He was coherent and lucid. We discussed the issues of tolerance to morphine. I suggested that dose increases were not due to tolerance but rather to disease progression. I encouraged him to accurately report any breakthrough pain so we could find the correct dose to keep him comfortable. A family conference was organised with Max, his daughter, nursing staff, the general practitioner and myself. It was agreed that quality of life was now the aim. The aged care facility was able to commit itself to having Max stay there, as professional nursing staff were available from the nursing home on site 24 hours a day.

A good palliative care order was completed by the GP for keeping in the clinical record. The order is a South Australian attempt to go past the 'do not resuscitate' orders of the past and rather to focus on what can be done to maintain or increase quality of life. It is not legally binding but formalises discussions between the doctor, resident (if appropriate), relatives and other staff, where active versus palliative care has been discussed. This ensures that all involved have the same goals and can be used to dissuade locum doctors who want to transfer residents to hospital after hours, as sometimes happens. The following issues were also discussed:

- Subcutaneous infusion of opioid analgesics (with or without a sedative) when necessary, to relieve pain and distress.
- Dehydration issues. Max will need diligent mouth care as a dry mouth is the main symptom of dehydration.
- A palliative focus now, rather than curative, for wound care. The wound was now left moistened with hydrogel and loose dressing

only. It was dressed every second day rather than twice daily, with no aim of debriding.

Soon after, a subcutaneous infusion of 80 mg morphine, 40 mg maxalon every 24 hours was commenced. The dose of morphine was increased over the next two weeks to 140 mg and Max was drowsy but easily roused and reported a satisfactory level of comfort. Despite being more comfortable, he still was definite about his decision. Max did take very small amounts of fluids over this time. The majority of staff did not press Max to drink, although some staff found this difficult and needed to be discouraged from pressing him to drink, so that Max's wishes could be met. Max's nausea abated as he took less food and fluids. Max died 18 days after his initial decision was voiced to staff. Four days before he died, 5 mg of midazolam (a sedative) was added to the morphine and maxalon, as he was becoming restless and agitated. Max was unconscious for only the last two days.

I followed up by debriefing with relevant staff the day after Max's death. The staff vented a lot of feelings about their helplessness, and frustration that Max had not died of a life-threatening condition, rather a conscious effort on his part to die by starvation. However, they felt it was made easier because they felt well supported throughout the whole process. I called Helen, Max's daughter, the next day and spoke at length with her. It is routine to then refer the relatives to the bereavement program of our palliative care service.

legislation relating to palliative care

Each state has its own legislative requirements relating to choices of treatment at the end of life. However, everyone has a common law right to refuse treatment and not to be assaulted. It is also possible for family members to make some medical decisions on behalf of an incompetent patient.

In NSW, individuals can appoint one or more people as 'enduring guardians' with the legal authority to make substitute decisions on their behalf. This means that it is possible to appoint someone who will have the legal authority to refuse unwanted medical treatment. The combination of both an enduring guardian and an advance directive gives legal weight to the patient's wishes. Each state has its own sets of criteria and you will need to check these with your Guardianship Tribunal or similar body.

The good palliative care order form in Appendix 11.1 was produced after the South Australian *Consent to Medical Treatment and Palliative Care Act 1995*. It is not the only form that can be used to document an agreement for palliative care in writing; however, it is an excellent Australian example of a suitable form of covenant between care staff and the resident and/or family about ongoing care for a patient

This form is designed to be reviewed at regular intervals. The most sensible practice is to discuss arrangements early in the care of an older person. Since today's emphasis in aged care is so heavily orientated to keeping a person at home, it is the primary responsibility of the coordinator of the community care program to ensure that this kind of directive is completed, discussed and updated regularly. If a person has not received community care then this kind of directive can be filled in when they enter an aged care facility. Once again, a system of reviewing the order at least three monthly, and after any acute episode, needs to be rigorously maintained.

The stickers mentioned in the recommendations in Appendix 11.1 are available from the Palliative Care Council of SA, but it would be quite possible to make your own. It is also possible to use a form such as the one in Appendix 11.2, which is issued by the World Federation of Right-to-Die Societies and is an agreed generic that can be used throughout the world.

In cases where an elderly family member is suffering from dementia and is drawing close to death, the strains on the family are often overwhelming. If the family members are not in agreement regarding treatment options, and no advanced directive is in place, it is frequently too late at this point to sort out a clear palliative plan. However, where possible, this is a situation to be managed, not one that can be used to abrogate the responsibility of assisting people with their choice to have a dignified death.

There have been numerous court cases where one part of a family has challenged another over their right to make a decision to 'let a person die'. There have also been cases where a hospital has challenged the right of a family, for example, to have artificial feeding ceased. These cases are the ones that make sensational news stories. Rather than letting these cases paralyse change, implementing well documented procedures and using skilled nursing diagnosis and communication will safely manage all but the exceptional case.

assessing and managing symptoms

Symptom assessment and treatment for palliative care for older people needs a different approach to assessment for a person with cancer, for example. This chapter will not deal with palliative care for cancer, in particular, as there are many referenced sources for that care. Instead, concentration will be on palliative care for older people with chronic conditions:

diagnosis

Firstly, the diagnosis must be quite clear. For example, a person with advanced, chronic obstructive airways disease is not going to be cured, neither is a person with irreversible dementia. These are terminal illnesses, just as certain forms of cancer are. Therefore, the diagnosis needs to be very clear. Once a diagnosis of an irreversible condition has been made, then working towards a palliative care plan can be a sensible approach. The way in which this is undertaken will depend on the patient's or the patient's family's values, beliefs, education, socioeconomic status, coping abilities and a myriad of other factors. With a clear philosophy, educated practitioners and good will, a palliative care plan can be achieved. Treatment of symptoms can then be assessed from the view of the comfort and quality of life of the patient rather than attempting to cure the underlying cause.

symptom control

The philosophy of hospice care—'no rush; no rules'—can still be the first choice in care for residents who need comfort, when they can't be cured. The principle of planning for what might happen is exactly the same in the case of palliative care for the older person as it is in any other palliative care approach.

Figure 11.1 shows the kind of lower limb breakdown that is seen in many older patients. If this is to be assessed for curative purposes, then the approach is not the same as being assessed for palliation. For example, would this person be more comfortable, and in less pain, if she had a soothing cream on her legs, and a stockinet covering, rather than butterflies to hold the wounds together, covered by ordinary nylon stockings? Here are some ideas to assist in assessing how to deal with body breakdown and implementing palliation:

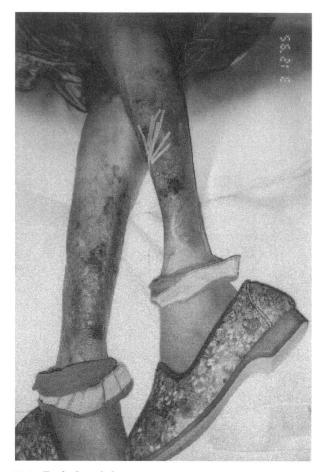

Figure 11.1: Body breakdown

- Keep information about products current by ensuring regular contact
  with and information from suppliers, following research and reading
  product reviews. Differentiate between those products that are
  designed for comfort and those that are designed for cure.
- Think about using procedures to ensure comfort, for example:
  - hot towel baths rather than a shower
  - bandages rather than sticking plaster
  - sheepskins, heel protectors, adjustable chairs.
- Decide, and document, when leaving someone in bed is more
  comfortable than getting them out.

• Decide, and document, when turning in bed may be more painful and discomforting than the development of pressure sores and stiffness.

treatments

The technical training of nursing staff seems to lead to the medical or clinical model of care being the automatic, and therefore comfortable, response to dying. The position taken instinctively is that you are doing your job 'right' if you are doing what you were taught. When a chest infection ensues, suction, antibiotics and breathing exercises feel right when someone is looking distressed, usually because there is no alternative planned palliative care. Suction must be a terrible experience; an alternative may be to assess whether the following may be more comfortable:

• reduce fluids drastically
• give medication to dry secretions, and
• give pain relief (assess, for example, if nebulised morphine may be useful).

I have documented many cases where nurses are valiantly attempting to give people antibiotics in the days before they die. Giving antibiotics is also the usual response to a urinary tract infection, but some alternatives to be assessed may be:

• to increase fluids, if this is comfortable for the patient
• to give pain relief, especially aspirin, if there is a fever
• to offer cranberry juice to drink.

For 15 residents with late-stage dementia who were studied in the last 12 to 18 months of their life, all but one received multiple doses of antibiotics over the course of their last years. The average number of courses during their stay in a nursing home was six (Abbey, 1995). The question of routine administration of antibiotics in nursing homes has been questioned by many for some time. For example, Yoshikawa and Norman (1994, p. 84) say:

> ... [the ageing of the population] behoves us to address the problem of infections and the use of antimicrobials in NHs [Nursing Homes] ... We must look at the problem as a multi-faceted one, viewing it not only from the microbiological perspective, but also from an ethical, societal, and financial viewpoint, since limited resources may force the medical profession into a triage situation of rationing care to those most likely to benefit from it.

> ... When a patient is admitted to a NH, it is imperative that the
> patient's physician (and the NH physician if they are separate
> individuals) explain in a compassionate but detailed manner the
> choices that a patient and/or family must face in terms of advanced
> directives, living will, and durable power of attorney for health care.

Since the administration of antibiotics is the most frequent treatment
prescribed to deal with acute conditions in older people with chronic illnesses, it is the one I have focused on; however, pre-planning for such
issues as treatment of fractures, transient ischaemic attacks (TIAs), fits
and heart failure, is an essential part of palliation. It may be that calling
the doctor or the ambulance may be in the best interests of the facility
and the peace of mind of the nurse-in-charge, but is it in the best interests of the patient? This does not mean that fractures and so on are
ignored or left undiagnosed for days, as I have seen documented on
many occasions, rather that if a fracture, heart failure or TIA is suspected,
a planned palliative treatment plan is put into place.

pain

Pain is a warning system, often the first sign that the body is out of
balance, that something is going wrong, and the damaged or stressed
cells are releasing the prostaglandins that trigger pain receptors. Pain
can also be due to emotional causes—we speak of 'the pain of separation' for example—or from inner frustration and rage with life. For older
people with chronic illnesses, especially for people with dementia, this
internal anger may be magnified. The terms 'suffering' and 'distress' can
cover the vast amount of ground there is between these two simple
explanations for pain. The literature that relates to pain and the elderly,
in particular pain and dementia, is peppered with comments about how
little is known about the subject, how difficult it is to diagnose and how
complex the process is. All this is true; however, it is not very helpful to
the practitioner.

As people become older, the prospect of pain, lack of mobility
and loss of dignity are their greatest fears. A clinical, linear approach
will not help you assist clients who now confront an adjustment to
just this situation. The eight-step problem-solving model illustrated in
Chapter 1 helps the assessor to think through this complex situation to
derive relevant person-centred care. A framework where pain and suffering is measured provides security to a health professional, since judgments can be based on notions of proof and evidence. We do not have
the luxury of that proof. Suffering, distress and pain for chronically ill

older people has not been measured in any way that is universally accepted. Some attempts have been made to provide tools to do this but these are early models that have many limits. Complicating the matter further is the fact that it has been shown that different health professionals work under very distinct paradigms of care and this can lead to friction and tension (Abbey, 1995). Research has also shown that there are distinct differences between clients' perceptions of care, what they want from it and what they get, and those of case managers. It has also been found that care givers 'engage in suffering-denying behaviours and use platitudes and reassurances to avoid the experience' (McCullough and Wilson, 1995, p. 246) of coping with dying.

The diagnosis and treatment of pain cannot be removed from how worrying it is for you, as the direct service provider, to be sure that your assessment is correct, or that your handling of the situation can be defended. Many studies that measure physical pain relief, especially in relation to the elderly and the use of narcotics, find that control is inadequate. The main reasons seem to be that the myths about respiratory depression and addiction still persist, but equally important is that pain relief is not given a high priority in case management for elderly people. So, the most important thing to do before we start talking about pain management is to say: 'put pain on the agenda'.

Always consider that pain may be present. As one author puts it, 'Recognising the increased risk of pain in old age, nurses must assume that pain is present until proven otherwise' (Parke, 1992, p. 93).

links between pain and depression

There is evidence that the links between chronic pain and depression in older people are strong. It is known that the way an individual interprets their situation, how much control they have or how they are coping will greatly influence their emotional states and behavioural responses (Turk, Okifiyi and Scharff, 1995). We also know that people who are assured that the future they face will be one where they feel cared for and comfortable, will be less depressed, and this is even more so if the future they face is certain death.

Here are some suggestions about questions to find out if pain is present. Many of the answers do not depend on the person's cognition being intact, as they rely on observation and holistic assessment.

- Ask, 'Are you in pain?' Use a pain chart to assist in pinpointing the type and extent of the pain.

- Has there been a change in behaviour? For example, has the person become aggressive, or, from being an outgoing person have they become quiet and withdrawn? Have they stopped wanting to do things (eg, have a shower) that they did not mind doing previously?
- Has there been a change in sleeping pattern?
- Are they guarding any part of their body?
- Has there been a change in appetite?
- Has there been a change in activity (eg, more or less walking)?
- Are there any obvious physical signs that could indicate pain (eg, chest rattles, skin tears, inflamed ear drum, cyanosis)?
- Are they exhibiting non-verbal cues; for example, frowning, grimacing, groaning, whimpering, screwing up their eyes, crying, hitting out (especially when moved)?
- Has there been a distressing event in their life recently (eg, loss of a pet)?
- Has there been a change in bowel habits (eg, voiding more often, constipation, diarrhoea)?
- Has there been any change in medication?
- Has the person vomited or seemed nauseous?
- Are they perspiring and/or have they got a temperature?
- Are they exhibiting pain by their body movements (eg, rocking, pulling legs up to the stomach, pacing, picking at bedclothes, moving the head from side to side)?
- Is the person verbally expressing pain (eg, 'it hurts') or in any way that could be interpreted as pain (eg, 'help me' or 'mummy, mummy')?

Once the presence of pain has been assessed, then treatment may take many forms (eg, massage, heat, transcutaneous electrical nerve stimulation (TENS) and analgesics). The effects of all treatments will then need to be further assessed (eg, if morphine is a chosen analgesic then a well known side effect is constipation, which will, in turn, need to be treated for comfort purposes). If the person has dementia, judging the effects of pain relief is more difficult, but hopefully, the pain scale for people with dementia who cannot verbalise, that is presently being tested and validated (Abbey et al., 1999) will assist.

nutrition and hydration

Steiner and Bruera (1998, p. 6) state that:

> A strong and often polarised debate has taken place during recent
> years concerning the consequences of dehydration in the terminally
> ill patient. When a patient has a severely restricted oral intake or is
> found to be dehydrated, the decision to administer fluids should be
> individualised and made on the basis of a careful assessment that
> considers problems related to dehydration, potential risks and
> benefits of fluid replacement, and patients' and families' wishes.

The question of sustenance is emotionally charged and causes great
concern for care workers. Issues such as incontinence, for example—the
other end of the sustenance chain—although distressing and the 'dirty
work' of caring for older people, are often simple in contrast. The
task is clear and unequivocal. You clean up the person and make them
comfortable. There is satisfaction in a job well done.

A palliative care protocol can include guidelines for withdrawal of
food and fluid that are acceptable to staff and family and would be comfortable for the dying resident. However, this needs to be set within a
context, as outlined by Lynne (1989, p. 176):

> Forgoing food and water must not become a thoughtless choice
> aimed at ridding society—or the patients' families—of burdensome,
> dependent elderly persons. Since the history of decision making in
> long-term facilities shows many deficiencies, procedures for deciding
> about nutrition and hydration should arise from a deliberate process
> and should be explicit and carefully evaluated in practice.

Some advantages of dehydration for the dying patient can be that
lower urinary output will assist in comfort because of the need for fewer
uncomfortable procedures (eg, when sheets are changed). Pulmonary
secretions decrease, which may result in less coughing, shortness of
breath and congestion. Dehydration can also assist in the reduction of
nausea, vomiting and abdominal pain. Some disadvantages are a dry
mouth and, sometimes, an electrolyte imbalance that can lead to muscle
spasms and contribute to an altered level of consciousness. A dry mouth
can be treated by giving the person ice chips if their swallowing reflex
is still intact or by regular mouth toilets. The problem of muscle spasms
can be treated with antispasmodics or sedation. A change of consciousness, where the person slips into a moribund state, can lead to a
peaceful and pain-free death.

This condition is characterised in its early stages by the person being thirsty, but the administering of small amounts of water may actually worsen rather than lessen the symptoms. Eventually, terminally ill patients will present with mixed disorders of salt and water depletion. Billings (1985, p. 108) says that:

> Disorders of thirst and the mental status changes that foster and perpetuate salt and water deficiencies may protect against discomfort or obliterate the awareness of suffering. Indeed, patients who become dehydrated may be too lethargic to be troubled by symptoms potentially produced by fluid deprivation.

Billings (ibid., p. 109) concludes that fluid depletion in dying patients is best dealt with by mouth care only; any administration of fluids is more often 'determined by the symbolic or emotional meanings of such measures'.

conclusion

Assessing the need for and implementation of palliative care for elderly people with chronic terminal illness is problematic; there is no point in avoiding this. It is a challenge to the sensitivity, compassion and professional integrity of the nurse caring for the person and interacting with the family. On the other hand, assisting a person to die in comfort and dignity, and to leave the family with the feeling that the death was a good one is, perhaps, the ultimate in nursing service to patients and the community.

study questions

1   What is meant by palliative care?
2   Reflect on the philosophy of where you work and relate the definition of palliative care to the values expressed in the philosophy of your workplace. Do they match?
3   Discuss the necessity of objective assessment that reinforces the decisions made in palliative care.

references

Abbey, J. (1995), 'Death and dementia in institutions, A cultural analysis', unpublished doctoral thesis.

Abbey, J., Giles, L., Piller, N., De Bellis, A., Gaston, J., Mitchell, J. and Parker, D. (1999), 'A pain scale for people with dementia who cannot say "it hurts"', paper submitted for the Alzheimer's conference, Perth, WA, September.

Billings, J. (1985), 'Comfort measures for the terminally ill. Is dehydration painful?', Editorial, *Journal of the American Geriatrics Society*, November, 33(11), pp. 808–10.

Charlesworth, M. (1993), *Bioethics in a Liberal Society*, Cambridge University Press, Cambridge.

Jacques, A. (1992), *Understanding Dementia*, 2nd edn, Churchill Livingstone, Edinburgh.

Jenkins, P. 'Case study: Palliative care assessment in the aged care setting', CNC Southern Hospice Unit, Repatriation Hospital, South Australia.

Kuhse, H. (ed.) (1994), *Willing to Listen, Wanting to Die*, Penguin Books, Melbourne.

Lowden, B. (1998), 'Research study. Introducing palliative care: Health professionals' perceptions', *International Journal of Palliative Nursing*, May-Jun, 4(3), pp. 135–42.

Lynne, J. (ed.) (1989), *By No Extraordinary Means. The Choice to Forgo Life-sustaining Food and Water*, Indiana University Press, Bloomington.

McCullough, L. and Wilson, N. (eds) (1995), *Long-Term Care Decisions, Ethical and Conceptual Dimensions*, The Johns Hopkins University Press, Baltimore.

MacMahon, D. G. and Thomas, S. (1998), 'Practical approach to quality of life in Parkinson's disease: The nurse's role', *Journal of Neurology*, May, 245 Suppl. 1, pp. S19–22.

O'Boyle, C. A. and Waldron, D. (1997), 'Quality of life issues in palliative medicine', *Journal of Neurology*, Oct, 244 Suppl. 4, pp. S18–25.

Parke, B. (1992), 'Pain in the cognitively impaired elderly', *Canadian Nurse*, 88(7), pp. 17–20.

Royal College of Nursing, Australia (1995), *Euthanasia, An Issue for Nurses. Discussion Paper No. 1*, Royal College of Nursing, Australia, Canberra.

Singer, P. (1994), *Rethinking Life and Death*, The Text Publishing Company, Melbourne.

Starck, P. L. (1992), 'The management of suffering in a nursing home: An ethnographic study' in P. C. Starck and J. P. Mc Govern (eds), *The Hidden Dimension of Illness: Human Suffering*, National League for Nursing Press, New York.

Steiner, N. and Bruer, E. (1998), 'Methods of hydration in palliative care patients', *Journal of Palliative Care*, Summer, 14(2), pp. 6–13.

Tonti-Filippini, N. (1994), 'Euthanasia undermines rights of sick', Opinion, *The Australian*, July 20, p. 11.

Turk, D. C., Okifiyi, A. and Scharff, L. (1995), 'Chronic pain and depression: Role of perceived impact and perceived control in different age cohorts', *Pain*, 61, pp. 93–101.

Yoshikawa, T. and Norman, D. (1994), *Antimicrobial Therapy in the Elderly Patient*, Marcel Dekker Inc, New York.

Appendix 11.1: Good palliative care order form

The Palliative Care Council of South Australia has surveyed professional attitudes to the concept of Good Palliative Care Orders, which were suggested for implementation in South Australia by the Parliamentary Select Committee on the Law and Practice Relating to Death and Dying.

A Reference Group of the Council, chaired by Professor Ian Maddocks, has prepared a report for the Council based on the survey findings, and has included the following recommendations which have been forwarded to the South Australian Health Commission, the Universities and Centres for Post Graduate Education, and all Hospitals and Nursing Homes throughout the State.

Recommendations

1 *Palliative Care education programs should be implemented.*

   The findings of the survey have highlighted a number of areas where education could improve current practice. These include:
   * the need for multidisciplinary consultation in the area of palliative care and, to that end, education with a multidisciplinary focus;
   * the need for education for junior medical staff to enable them to feel more confident in discussing issues surrounding death and dying with their patients and those patients' families;
   * the provision of information to all medical and nursing staff concerning the laws which relate to medical treatment and, more specifically, death and dying.

2 *Hospitals and Nursing Homes should adopt policies regarding Good Palliative Care and should implement procedures for Good Palliative Care Orders and Anticipatory Directions.*

   The attached document incorporates the concepts of Good Palliative Care and is an example of such an Order, designed to be included in patient case notes. A sticker has also been designed and it is suggested that this be placed on the front of the case notes to indicate the presence of an Order in the notes, and the need to consult it.

   The Palliative Care Council recommends that copies of this form and the accompanying sticker should be available for use in all hospitals and nursing homes, together with the following instructions about how to complete the form.

Instructions

Clearly fill in the name of the patient for whom a Good Palliative Care Order-Anticipatory Direction is indicated, having discussed the issues involved with them, their family and other staff as appropriate.

Under the Consent to Medical Treatment and Palliative Care Act 1995, a person can appoint a medical agent to make decisions for them if they are unable to make decisions for themselves. The agent must produce proof of agency before assuming control of medical decisions.

Appendix 11.1: (continued)

Include the names of family members and staff members who have been involved in discussions regarding the patient's condition and future care plan.

Under the Guardianship and Administration Act 1993 family members are able to make medical decisions should there not be a guardian or medical agent. A family member includes spouse, official de facto, parent, child over eighteen, and sibling over eighteen.

Describe the patient's condition and likely prognosis.

Identify if the patient is competent, that is, able to make decisions regarding their medical care.

Under the Consent to Medical Treatment and Palliative Care Act, patients can also write down their wishes regarding their future medical care which come into effect only if they are not able to make decisions regarding that care. Once sighted these documents, called anticipatory directions or advance directives, must be followed.

Select the option which best conforms to the patient's, or delegate's, desire for future medical treatment. Should none of the three written options be appropriate, provision is made for specific instruction under point four.

Identify how long you wish this document to be in force for and when you believe that it should be reviewed.

Date the document, sign it and clearly print your name. This document should be signed by a medical practitioner. It is expected that the care team will be consulted as part of its completion.

If using the accompanying sticker to indicate the existence of the Order in the notes, affix it to the front of the case notes and note the date the Order is completed.

Appendix 11.1: (continued)

Good Palliative Care Order Form

Anticipatory Direction

I have discussed with patient

or with their medical agent

Please ensure the medical power of attorney, authorising the agent, is sighted.

and/or family members or attending persons

and with staff members

the patient's current condition, which can be described as

The patient is competent ○
incompetent ○
The patient has made an anticipatory direction which has been sighted
Yes ○   No ○

Circle one of the options

We have agreed that in the event of further deterioration in the patient's condition

1   Full cardiopulmonary resuscitation with total body support as required will be undertaken

2   Intensive medical support will be undertaken, but cardiopulmonary resuscitation will not be initiated, and no long-term support measures, including ventilation or dialysis, will be undertaken.

3   The emphasis of management will be on Good Palliative Care, highlighting the relief of symptons and discomforts. No artificial measures designed to supplant or support bodily function will be undertaken.

4   Other. Please specify

This form will be in force for
1 week ○ 1 month ○ 3 months ○
12 months ○ indefinitely ○
or until revoked by the patient ○

Date

Signed

Print name of legally qualified medical practitioner

Appendix 11.2: Living will

This document should be lodged with the declarant's medical records.

A doctor having conscientious objection should immediately refer the declarant to another doctor. Living wills are accepted by common law. The form does not ask the doctor to do anything illegal. Duplicate copies may optionally be lodged with a solicitor or close friend and a further copy kept for reference.

section a. advance medical directive

- **Note:** This section may be legally binding.
- Section A comprises specific instructions to the health care team in the event that I can no longer express my own wishes; it covers very serious conditions.
- **To the declarant:** When filling out this part of the form, you should cross out anything that does not express your true wishes, then initial any changes clearly.

section b. life values statement

This gives indications of the personal value I attach to my life under various circumstances. I ask my health care team to bear these in mind when making difficult decisions about my treatment or non-treatment, especially in situations not covered by Section A. Where I have indicated that life under such circumstances would be 'much worse than death' this means that I would find the situation totally unbearable and unacceptable, and that I would prefer all life-sustaining treatment to be stopped or withdrawn rather than exist for the rest of my life in such a state.

Note: A doctor should not be liable to civil or criminal proceedings if she or he acts in good faith and with reasonable care in respecting the directives and values in this document.

DO NOT FILL OUT THIS FORM WITHOUT DEEP AND CAREFUL CONSIDERATION.

Complete Section A or Section B or both.

This living will form was developed by C. G. Docker and is © 1994, revised 1996. Requests for reprinting are welcomed, however; together with suggestions for further development which should be addressed to C. G. Docker, BM 718, London WC1N 3XX, U.K. Much of the text is drawn from existing documents, and many individuals and organisations have contributed ideas and made helpful suggestions, including the National Agency for Welfare and Health, Helsinki and the Ethics Committee of the Seattle Veterans Affairs Medical Center.

Personal copies may be made by the Declarant for his or her own use.

section a. advance medical directive

To my physician and health care team, my family, my solicitor and all other persons concerned: this declaration is made at a time when I am of sound mind and after careful consideration.

Appendix 11.2: (continued)

I understand that my life may be shortened by the specific refusals of treatment made in this document.

I declare that if at any time the following circumstances exist, namely:

1 I suffer from one or more of the conditions mentioned in the *Schedule*; and
2 I have become unable to participate effectively in decisions about my medical care; and
3 two independent physicians (one a consultant) are of the expert, considered opinion, after full examination of my case, that I am unlikely to make a substantial recovery from illness or impairment involving severe distress or incapacity for rational existence,

then and in those circumstances my directions are as follows:

1 that I am not to be subjected to any medical intervention or treatment (aimed at prolonging my life) such as life support systems, artificial ventilation, antibiotics (ie, to control infection), artificial feeding—whether enteral or parenteral (tube feeding into the stomach or into a vein), invasive surgery, dialysis (eg, using a kidney machine), or blood transfusion;
2 that any distressing symptoms (including any caused by lack of food or fluid) are to be fully and aggressively controlled by appropriate palliative care, ordinary nursing care, analgesic or other treatments, even though some of these treatments may have the secondary effect of shortening my life.

However, modes of treatment mentioned in (1) above may be applied for elimination of serious symptoms. Giving intensive care to me is to be allowed only on the condition that reliable reasons exist for the possibility that such treatment will have a better result than merely short prolongation of life. In the event that a treatment with prospect of recovery has been started but proves to be futile, it has to be discontinued immediately.

I consent to anything proposed to be done or omitted in compliance with the directions expressed above and absolve my medical attendants from any civil liability arising out of such acts or omissions.

I offer the health care team my heartfelt thanks for respecting my sincerely held wishes, as expressed in this directive.

I accept the risk that I may be unable to express a change of mind at a time in the future when I am incapacitated, that improving medical technology may offer increased hope, but I personally consider the risk of unwanted treatment to be a greater risk. *I wish it to be understood that I fear degradation and indignity far more than death.* I ask my medical attendants to bear this statement in mind when considering what my intentions would be in any uncertain situation.

I reserve the right to revoke this directive at any time, orally or in writing, but unless I do so, it should be taken to represent my continuing directions. I hereby deliberately accept the risk that I may no longer be able to revoke my declaration if I am in a condition listed in the Schedule, in order to exclude a risk which is greater to me, namely that I should continue living in circumstances that are not acceptable to me.

Appendix 11.2: (continued)

schedule

A   Advanced disseminated malignant disease (eg, cancer that has spread considerably).

B   Severe immune deficiency (eg, Acquired Immune Deficiency Syndrome).

C   Advanced degenerative disease of the nervous system (eg, advanced Parkinson's disease).

D   Severe and lasting brain damage due to injury, stroke, disease or other cause.

E   Advanced dementia, whether Alzheimer's, multi-infarct or other, resulting in very limited awareness of the immediate environment and inability to initiate simple tasks.

F   Any other condition of comparable gravity.

Additional instructions (if any, such as pregnancy waiver)
....
....
....

If you would like a particular person's wishes to be taken into consideration during decisions about your medical care, please give their details here:
Name of my proxy ....
Telephone number ....
Address ....
....

To my proxy: Please try to ensure that decisions are taken:
(mark one box only)   ☐   how you believe I would have taken them
                                 ☐   using your own best judgment.

I have discussed this document with my doctor   ☐ (Mark here if yes)

No

Name of Doctor ....

Doctor's telephone number ....

Address ....

It is not obligatory to discuss your living will in advance with your doctor, but it may be very helpful to do so.

Appendix 11.2: (continued)

section b. values history statement

Please use this section as a guide to my values when considering the likely result of treatment.

Circle the number on the scale of one to five, that most closely indicates your feelings about each of the situations described	Much worse than death: I would definitely not want life-sustaining treatment	Somewhat worse than death: I would probably not want life-sustaining treatment	Neither better nor worse than death: I'm not sure whether I want life-sustaining treatment	Somewhat better than death: I would probably want life-sustaining treatment	Much better than death: I would definitely want life-sustaining treatment
(a) Permanently paralysed. You are unable to walk but can move around in a wheelchair. You can talk and interact with other people.	1	2	3	4	5
(b) Permanently unable to speak meaningfully. You are unable to speak to others. You can walk on your own, feed yourself and take care of daily needs such as bathing and dressing yourself.	1	2	3	4	5
(c) Permanently. unable to care for yourself. You are bedridden, unable to wash, feed, or dress yourself. You are totally cared for by others.	1	2	3	4	5
(d) Permanently in pain. You are in severe bodily pain that cannot be totally controlled or completely eliminated by medications.	1	2	3	4	5
(e) Permanently mildly demented. You often cannot remember things, such as where you are, nor reason clearly. You are capable of speaking, but not capable of remembering the conversations; you are capable of washing, feeding and dressing yourself and are in no pain.	1	2	3	4	5
(f) Being in a short-term coma. You have suffered brain damage and are not conscious and are not aware of your environment in any way. You cannot feel pain. You are cared for by others. These mental impairments may be reversed in about one week leaving mild forgetfulness and loss of memory as a consequence.	1	2		4	5

Appendix 11.2: (continued)

Signature of declarant to Sections A & B: ....

Name (print clearly) ....

Day/Month/Year ....

Address ....

Date of Birth* ....

*If you are under 18 years of age, you may still complete this document, though it may not have the same legal force.

Witness's signature: I declare that the above named has signed this document in my presence. He/she has declared it to be his/her firm will, is in full capacity and fully understands the meaning of it. I believe it to be a firm and competent statement of his/her wishes. As far as I am aware, no pressure has been brought to bear on him/her to sign such a document and I believe it to be his/her own free and considered wish. So far as I am aware, I do not stand to gain from his/her death.

Signed (Witness) ....

Name ....

Address ....

The Voluntary Euthanasia Society of Scotland, January 1995. Reproduced with permission.

Appendix 11.3: Some guidance notes on completing your living will

(These notes do not form part of the living will document.)

Note: If you are admitted to hospital with a serious illness, you are strongly advised to ask for your living will so that you can review it, update it, or affirm that it still represents your current wishes.

It is not necessary generally to insert any additional instructions on your living will, but the following are exceptions that certain people may wish to consider. If you are adding any wording in the 'additional instructions' section, it is advisable to discuss it thoroughly with a doctor first.

example 1: dementia declaration

Your living will already recognises the extreme forms of senile dementia—situations where you do not recognise your nearest relations, no longer know the time in which you live, and are no longer capable of performing the activities of daily life such as eating, drinking, washing, going to the toilet. If you also want to emphasise that you refuse treatment in the *initial* phase of senile dementia, which is characterised by periods of extreme confusion, interspersed with periods of extreme lucidity, you can add: 'In the event that I find myself in the situation of the beginning of senile dementia and also have a life-threatening physical condition, I refuse all further life-sustaining treatment'.

example 2: declaration of non-resuscitation

One of the natural ways by which a lasting suffering can be ended is a cardiac arrest. A person to whom this happens is unconscious immediately. If no immediate action is taken, the patient will die within a short time, dying a fairly mild death. When a cardiac arrest occurs, however, health care teams would generally make attempts to resuscitate the patient as soon as possible. These can take the form of heart massage, mouth-to-mouth resuscitation, or more sophisticated measures. Resuscitation, however, is undesirable if you consider cardiac arrest as a relief or if, in view of your age or medical condition, you consider the chances of complete recovery after resuscitation to be very small. Your doctor should be able to give you information about the eventual consequences of resuscitation in your situation.

If you do not want resuscitation, you will have to talk this over in good time with your doctor, your family, social workers or those close to you. You will have to consider very carefully if your wish for non-resuscitation applies to all circumstances. The following text, which also includes accident and drowning, could be added to your living will for non-resuscitation, but should *only* be included after discussion with your doctor: 'I refuse all life-sustaining treatment in case I find myself in a situation of unconsciousness caused by cardiac arrest, accident or drowning. I also refuse any draining of my stomach.'

Appendix 11.3: (continued)

example 3: pregnancy waiver/non-waiver

If you are a woman of child-bearing age, you may wish to consider whether your wishes about non-treatment should apply if you were carrying a viable fetus. You could then add one of the following texts:

- 'This living will is to be temporarily overruled if I am pregnant and, to a reasonable degree of medical certainty, the fetus may develop to the point of live birth.'
  or

- 'My advance refusal of treatment, as stated in this document, is to be carried out even if I am pregnant and carrying a viable fetus, and even if this means that the fetus will not develop to the point of a live birth.'

example 4: refusal of specific treatments

If you have a condition such as AIDS or multiple sclerosis, where the prognosis involving incapacity is known with some certainty, as are the available treatment options, you may wish to make advance refusals of specific treatments, such as chemotherapy, where there is likely to be a choice between benefits and burdens. If this is the case, suitable wording should be devised with your doctor and added to your living will.

what to say to your doctor

When you approach your doctor or medical consultant in order to lodge your living will in your medical records, you may be unsure as to his or her reaction. If your doctor has not come across a living will before, he or she may need some reassurance from you as to what it is. Bear the following points in mind, or take a photocopy of the following paragraph with you:

(You could say . . .) *'The purpose of the living will document is to minimise the indignity or suffering that might ensue in the event of certain irreversible conditions, and to spare doctors and relatives the problem of trying to make difficult decisions on my behalf.'*

It does not ask the doctor or nurse to do anything contrary to existing law—in fact the law fully upholds the right of any patient to decline treatment, including life-sustaining treatment, and to receive analgesic drugs in quantities to relieve intolerable distress.

If the doctor has personal objections to accepting the document or making its existence known at such times as may be appropriate, then an alternative doctor should be recommended who may not have the same reservations.

If at all possible, it is extremely desirable to discuss the living will with your doctor. Ask for the medical terms and the implications of refusing treatment to be explained so that you fully understand what you are signing. This will also mean that your doctor will be more fully aware of your wishes if he or she has to make difficult decisions at a time when you are no longer able to speak for yourself.

Appendix 11.3: (continued)

If you still have further queries about your living will, you can send a large stamped, self-addressed envelope and a small donation to VESS, 17 Hart St, Edinburgh EHI 3RN (UK) requesting a Living Will Information Pack which provides further answers to common questions, as well as guidance on some of the difficult areas of law and medical ethics concerning such documents. Members of VESS can also obtain living will stickers for medical files, a document carrying case, a medical alert card to carry in a wallet, and update stickers to indicate that the document has been renewed every few years. Subscription to VESS costs £15 per year (Overseas residents: £30) and includes a regular and comprehensive newsletter, which keeps you informed of any changes in the law or practice of living wills.

The Voluntary Euthanasia Society of Scotland January, 1995. Reproduced with permission.

assessment of the vision and hearing function of residents in aged care facilities

Richard Osborn and Wendy-Mae Rapson

chapter summary

An increasing proportion of our population is people older than 60 years. Sensory loss, which includes vision and hearing problems, is known to be the second most common health problem for people in this age cohort. Therefore, we need to be more aware of how to promote their ability to live safely and independently.

Carers must develop a critical understanding of the most effective ways to identify people with sensory loss and to provide specific practical assistance in a supportive environment for the many older people who experience such loss.

objectives

After reading and reflecting on this chapter, you will be able to:

- define what is meant by sensory loss
- discuss the impact of sensory loss on older people, especially those in residential care settings
- analyse the impact of both cognitive impairment and sensory loss
- critique the accuracy of types of sensory loss assessment strategies

introduction

Both hearing and vision difficulties are very common in older people. Sensory loss is the second most prevalent condition (after arthritis) ex-perienced by older Australians (ABS, 1993). Estimates of hearing loss vary between 31 per cent and 87 per cent (Voeks et al., 1993; Ward et al., 1993). Vision loss estimates vary between 10 per cent and 25 per cent in the older population (Klein, Klein and Lee, 1996; Kirchner and Peterson, 1980). More than 80 per cent of residents in nursing homes experience vision or hearing difficulties (Worral, Hickson and Dodd, 1993).

A vision or hearing impairment can have a serious impact on people's lives. It can affect their ability to walk about safely, to read, to recognise faces, to watch television, to talk on the telephone and to listen to the radio. Consequently, sensory loss may reduce a person's mobility and ability to communicate with family and friends. This can lead to with-drawal from enjoyable family, social and community activities, and force a loss of independence and quality of life. Many of the everyday tasks we engage in without thought or effort can become a significant burden for an older person with sensory loss.

Severe vision loss severely limits access to written communication and to important features of non-verbal aspects of speech. As the result of sensory loss, the ability to communicate effectively can be severely impaired, negatively affecting an older person's participation in everyday conversation. A vision or hearing loss can reduce the older person's participation in recreational and social activities such as those provided in many residential facilities and day programs. It often has a negative impact on the person's safety and security. Issues around compliance in taking medication, increased risk of falls, and social isolation that may compound any existing cognitive difficulties, are also associated with the presence of sensory loss. Every activity shared by care staff and the older person involves communication. Clear communication is essential for *all* areas of the older person's care and support, ranging from continence issues to the taking of medication and dining.

Fortunately, the negative impact that sensory loss has on people's lives is being appreciated by a far greater range of aged care providers. This chapter will describe the reliable, easily performed identification procedures, and a range of practical skills and strategies that carers need to develop to assist older people to manage more effectively with their sensory impairments. It is now a requirement for accreditation of residential care facilities that the sensory loss of residents is accurately assessed and that there are nursing plans in place that ensure residents' sensory aids and devices are adequately maintained and effectively used. In addition, residential care providers need to modify existing or provide new facilities to offer a less hostile environment for people with severe sensory loss.

Following the application of suitable design principles, residents with sensory loss can more confidently move about and safely conduct their daily activities. Also recommended is the installation of simple acoustic treatments and some audio equipment which enables residents to participate more fully in everyday conversation, which is so important for wellbeing and emotional health.

The impact of sensory loss on all aspects of daily living, and its effective management, must be understood and acted upon at all levels within the aged care sector. Training of aged care providers needs to include a far greater emphasis on the practical skills and support required by the many older people experiencing severe vision and/or hearing loss. Both initial training and continuing education programs must have greater content in the critical aspect of daily living needs, which is communication. Simulation experiences provide carers with greater insight into the needs of older people with sensory loss. They can also lead to a greater appreciation of how simple practical steps can help overcome some of the sensory difficulties experienced by most people in residential care. Carers must apply these practical strategies and promote positive intervention to encourage people to learn new ways of doing everyday tasks, thus maximising their independence and enhancing their quality of life.

assessment approaches

Because of the high prevalence of sensory loss in the older population, thorough individual assessment by an appropriate professional is strongly recommended every two years. Ophthalmologists, optometrists, ear, nose and throat specialists and audiologists can assess function, monitor changes, and recommend management and rehabilitation options. In our view, the clinical observations of experienced nurse practitioners working in aged care environments can be a valuable supplement to this process. Clients' observed behaviour, and their responses to questions about their sensory function, as well as the formal use of structured questionnaires, can guide the management of individuals' vision and hearing difficulties. Questions to guide assessment are listed in Appendix 12.1.

assessment rationale

It is important that residents have individual evaluation of their vision and hearing, to measure the extent of any loss and to describe appropriate intervention strategies to ensure their independent functioning is maximised. It is also critical to detect operable (eg, glaucoma, cataract, retinal detachment, otosclerosis, middle-ear effusion) or threatening conditions (eg, acoustic neuroma, cholesteotoma). There is also a duty of care to reduce secondary conditions such as the risk of falls due to vision or ear (balance) problems (Reinsch et al., 1992). In addition, we need to identify other factors of the person's health, lifestyle and environment which might compound any sensory loss. For example, the presence of severe arthritis in the hands or Parkinson's symptoms are going to effect a person's ability to independently manage a hearing aid or special reading magnifier. The cognitive function of the individual may also be a key issue. The existence of a significant degree of sensory loss may exacerbate an underlying dementia-related condition, and may even lead to misdiagnosis of cognitive and behavioural difficulties (McArdle, 1997). Certainly, the presence of dementia states make the clinical assessment of vision and hearing more challenging.

It is also important to routinely monitor older people's sensory functioning, since incremental changes can cause increasing difficulties, and aids and strategies that have worked effectively in the past may need to be updated to adjust to the new circumstances. In addition, new developments in technology may offer greater benefits to aid users, so regular reviews are recommended.

Accurate assessment also facilitates the development of effective and efficient care strategies and encourages specific goal setting and intervention plans. Individual rehabilitation plans include provision of information, counselling, planning of the visual and acoustic environment, supply of appropriate aids, training of skills and strategies, and assisting family members.

options for assessment

vision

The informed observation of residents' behaviour will provide the nurse practitioner with clear evidence of their functional ability in the area of visual performance (specific behaviours will be described below). In addition, self-reporting can be useful. However, the reliability of self-reported status is often questionable because of the slow onset of many conditions, the incremental adjustments that people make to their vision changes, the belief that such changes are an unavoidable aspect of old age, and a general lack of insight into their wellness.

Functional tests of visual function can also be used, such as standardised reading cards, assessing the person's ability to read magazines and newspaper articles (headlines, sub-headlines, text), and identifying people and objects in photographs. There are also standard vision handicap scales which can be used to identify older people with severe vision difficulties (Horowitz, Teresi and Cassels, 1991). In our experience, accurate observational assessment by experienced aged care practitioners offers a more robust option for identification.

hearing

Similar issues surround the assessment of hearing among older people. Again, the use of self-report approaches can be unreliable (Sanchez, Andrews and Boyd, 1998). Many people with significant hearing losses are unable or unwilling to acknowledge the degree of difficulty they experience in understanding what is being said. Informed observation of behaviour, such as leaning forward, cupping of the ear, requesting repetition of utterances, having the volume of the television or radio turned up loud, and using a loud voice, can provide the nurse practitioner with clues to identify those residents likely to have a significant hearing loss.

Functional tests of hearing function can also be used, such as standardised whisper tests (MacPhee, Crowther and McAlpine, 1988). Results are often affected by the stimulus material used, the level of stimulus presentation, the motivation of the older person being assessed, and by the acoustic environment in which the tests are conducted. Again, there are many standard hearing handicap scales that have been used to identify older people with severe hearing difficulties (Ventry and Weinstein, 1982; Schow and Nerbonne, 1982). In our experience, however, accurate observational assessment by experienced aged care practitioners provides the best means for identification.

vision

causes and effects of vision loss

It is important to understand the causes and effects of severe vision loss among older people. Very few residents are totally blind, but many experience severe vision difficulties due to the following conditions:

- Age-related macular degeneration (AMD) is the most common condition affecting older people. It produces a loss of central vision, leading to difficulty seeing detail, which affects the person's ability to read, recognise faces and perceive colour.
- Diabetic retinopathy produces a loss of parts of the visual field, causing a blurring and patchiness of vision, which affects safe movement, reading ability and the performance of many everyday activities.
- Glaucoma often produces a loss of peripheral vision, causing tunnel vision, which affects the person's ability to drive and move about safely.
- Cataracts produce a loss of contrast vision, causing blurring and increased glare sensitivity, which affects reading, face recognition and safe movement.

optical aids

When surgical and medical options have been exhausted, the person with these conditions requires assistance in the form of low vision aids and devices, training in their most effective use, learning new ways of performing everyday tasks, and support from family and carers.

Many people learn how to use specially prescribed optical aids to assist with near distance tasks (eg, using a hand-held illuminated magnifier for reading letters) and far distance tasks (eg, using a monocular for identifying street signs). Others may use adaptive devices such as talking books for reading material, or signature templates for signing cheques. Other such devices include needle-threaders, liquid-level indicators and talking clocks.

Learning new techniques often assists people to live with severe vision loss. The use of microwave ovens, reorganising the placement of objects in a room and pursuing new recreational activities may provide useful alternatives. Care providers can help maximise the person's independence by initially assisting in their learning of new skills and effective use of aids and devices.

vision assessment

Careful clinical measurement is necessary to describe an individual's impairment. Assessment of performance in three main areas of vision function—visual acuity, visual fields and contrast sensitivity—can be tested very simply by optometrists experienced in low vision assessment.

visual acuity difficulties

Visual acuity (the 'acuteness' of vision) can be measured using regular eye charts. In addition, visual acuity can be examined at non-standard test distances so that 'severe low vision' can be specified exactly by specialist optometrists. Behaviours in residents that indicate visual acuity difficulties, include:

- not recognising the faces of staff and relatives
- inability to follow the movement of an item of interest
- inability to see detail in objects, photos and magazines
- not seeing food on a plate
- spilling drinks or pouring difficulties
- inability to read, or enjoy television
- difficulty finding personal belongings (eg, on the bedside table)
- withdrawal from activities, such as bingo, that rely on vision
- gross eye signs such as rubbing of eyes, red or sore eyes, weeping eyes, and difference in pupil size.

visual field difficulties

The visual field refers to the panorama of vision, and is divided into central and peripheral visual functions. Peripheral visual field defects severely disable mobility. Special optical appliances can be used and alternative strategies for safe movement can be developed.

Behaviours that indicate visual field difficulties, include:

- bumping into furniture or other people
- disorientation within a room

- lack of confidence with mobility
- requiring much scanning of a room to see the objects within it
- withdrawal from group activities.

contrast sensitivity difficulties

Contrast sensitivity is the third major vision function. Simple clinical tests can be conducted by optometrists, which accurately specify this type of dysfunction. Sensitivity to contrast enables the detection of nuances of light and shade, and the ability to discriminate colour and contrast. Contrast sensitivity is essential for conducting many of the activities of daily living. Improve lighting and increase contrast between task objects eg, light wool on dark knitting needles.

Behaviours in residents that indicate contrast sensitivity difficulties include:

- failure to perceive differences in the colours of objects
- inability to discriminate the edges of objects (eg, plates, furniture, steps)
- inability to see clearly with normal levels of lighting.

support and assistance for vision impairment

Aged care providers can develop some useful strategies to support and assist older people with vision loss. Some simple but important strategies include:

- always introducing yourself
- asking whether the person requires assistance and how they would like to be helped
- learning sighted guide techniques (eg, offering your arm to be held)
- always putting objects back in their place
- providing verbal descriptions of the environment and activities taking place.

hearing

causes and effects of hearing loss

Understanding the nature and impact of age-related hearing loss is important for aged care providers, since good communication is essential to psychological wellbeing and independence. Presbycusis is the major cause of permanent sensori-neural hearing loss. For many people exposed to loud levels of industrial or recreational noise, an additional noise-induced component adds to the overall degree of their hearing loss. In general, a sensori-neural loss affects the perception of high-frequency sounds, and causes a reduction in the clarity of speech, particularly in noisy rooms or group conversations. Often sound distortion and increased sensitivity to loud sounds accompany hearing loss. Tinnitus, or a ringing sound in the ears, is also common. This type of hearing loss leads to difficulty following everyday conversation, especially group conversation and when there is background noise, and often results in the person withdrawing from social interaction.

hearing aids

As for vision loss, the use of aids is an effective way of reducing the difficulties experienced because of hearing loss. Fortunately, the performance of personal hearing aids has greatly improved in recent years. However, adapting to the different sound of the aid often requires some perseverance, and unrealistic expectations of fully restored hearing function may cause frustration for new wearers.

Other specialised hearing devices may be useful (eg, amplified telephones and television headphones). Actively assisting people to use these aids effectively and with confidence is an important component in adapting to living with a hearing loss.

hearing assessment

Audiological assessment generally involves determining the individual's hearing acuity across the range of speech frequencies. The nature of the loss will also be determined (ie, whether it is a sensori-neural ['nerve deafness'], conductive [mechanical dysfunction] or mixed loss). Speech discrimination ability will also be evaluated at a number of intensities to determine the amplification level at which speech understanding is maximised. The person's tolerance level for loud sounds will also be measured to ensure that aids do not generate sounds that are uncomfortably loud. The functioning of the outer and middle ear systems is assessed using impedance audiometry to help determine whether medical intervention may be indicated. This formal assessment will provide nursing staff with specific information about the hearing loss; its type, degree, and intervention options.

The aged care professional will observe behaviours in residents that indicate hearing difficulties, including:

- requesting frequent repetitions
- responding to conversation inconsistently
- complaining of 'people mumbling'
- startling at loud sounds
- having radio or television too loud.

Trained nursing staff can quickly and reliably screen whether an individual needs to be referred for a full hearing assessment. Parker and Osborn (1997) recommend a hearing screening test that involves the presentation of ten words from an AB word list (a common speech discrimination assessment tool) (Boothroyd, 1968) at a voice level of 60 dBA. If residents obtain a score of 8/10 correct or better, their hearing might be considered functionally adequate and immediate referral for audiological assessment is not indicated. If the resident gets less than 8/10 correct, it is likely that a hearing loss exists and referral for appropriate assessment should be made.

Another important assessment tool for nursing staff to evaluate hearing loss is observation of the resident during a conversation. Does the person:

- frequently request repetition
- give inappropriate responses
- lean forward and look confused or strained (due to the effort of trying to hear)
- have increased difficulty if there is background noise present
- perform better if amplification is used (eg, with their hearing aid or with an assistive listening device).

Does the person use hearing aids or an assistive listening device only for specific times of day? This is very important. A resident may not wish to use their hearing aid all of the time because of the background noise they will experience when not engaged in conversation. Nursing staff may need to know when the person uses their hearing aid or assistive listening device most effectively and encourage the person to use it at those times. Assistance with the insertion of the aid and its management may also be required.

support and assistance for hearing impairment

Aged care providers can also assist people with hearing impairments by developing some effective communication strategies, including:

- attracting the resident's attention before speaking
- avoiding or reducing background noise
- moving closer to the person when speaking to them
- speaking clearly and at a louder volume (but not shouting)
- using shorter sentences, with pauses between them
- having good lighting on your face to maximise lip-reading opportunities
- rephrasing or repeating messages that have not been understood
- using touch to focus the resident's attention, and for reassurance.

Further strategies for care planning are identified in Appendix 12.2.

the importance of well designed facilities

Facilities commonly used by older people, such as day centres, social venues and residential facilities, must be designed better to allow older people to move about and participate in activities more confidently. Simple actions such as providing better lighting, with minimal glare, and increasing the contrast between doors and the surrounding walls, can have a substantial effect. Similarly, the installation of acoustic and group audio equipment enables many people to participate more fully in everyday activities, including general group conversation.

Specifically, the following features should be considered in the design of facilities for vision and hearing impaired people:

- the size of rooms and the number of people in group activities (small groups; avoiding large rooms)
- sound reverberation in rooms should be reduced (absorption: carpet, curtains, tablecloths)
- internally-generated noise should be reduced (modification—dining room noise: use underlays, tablecloths and placemats to absorb sound; turn off televisions and radios)
- externally-generated noise should be reduced (location: traffic noise, isolation: plant noise; transmission: double-glazing)
- the level of speech signal should be increased through use of amplification: radio frequency sound system; microphones
- lighting (both natural and artificial) should be improved and glare reduced. This maximises use of residual lip-reading ability.

The quality of people's lives and their independence can be significantly improved, and at little cost, by applying some of these simple design principles. Other simple measures to assist people are to move closer to the person when speaking to them, and away from sources of noise, to close doors and windows, to turn off air conditioners, fountains, televisions and music, or to find a quieter room.

The difficulty experienced by vision impaired people in perceiving mouth movements cannot readily be overcome by modifications on the speaker's part. Lip-reading is an important part of communication when in presence of background noise. As this is not possible for many vision impaired people, it is important that the noise conditions be modified to ensure that these people are able to fully participate in activities and conversation (Erber and Osborn, 1994; Osborn et al., 2000). The provision of favourable listening conditions is particularly recommended in facilities that provide services for vision impaired people (eg, vocational and recreational centres, day centres and residential facilities). Group activities that are limited in size to four to six people will also be more satisfactory for people with vision and/or hearing difficulties.

case study: Margaret

Margaret is an 85-year-old woman who moved into a hostel residential setting because of a recent fracture and concerns of her family about her ability to live alone. Before moving, Margaret's main source of contact was with her family via the telephone and visits. Margaret was an avid reader but had been unable to read for a long while because of her deteriorating vision.

Margaret had age-related maculopathy and cataracts. Her family were greatly concerned because of her hearing loss—telephone conversations and face-to-face conversations had become increasingly difficult. Margaret presented as withdrawn and did not wish to participate in the hostel's social activities.

Several referrals were made upon Margaret's arrival. She was referred to a low vision clinic for assessment of her vision and to an audiologist for hearing tests. The nurse practitioner identified excessive ear wax and referral to Margaret's GP was made for its management.

At the end of these assessments, a moderate hearing loss was identified and Margaret was classified 'legally blind'. A hearing aid was recommended for conversation and group activities. Staff and family were instructed on how to use this, though the aim was for Margaret to use it independently. With amplification, Margaret was able to listen to talking books and she became a member of the talking book library. An amplified telephone with large numbers was obtained for Margaret to keep in touch with family and friends. With her ears clear of wax, the family reported better communication with Margaret.

The occupational therapist and activities director of the hostel aimed to find Margaret activities that would suit her social and sensory needs. Margaret agreed to go to the book reading group (a group which had amplification available) and to bingo twice a week where she used large print/tactile bingo cards. The occupational therapist also organised orientation and mobility training for Margaret so she could move about with confidence and ease in her new surroundings.

After three months, Margaret became a representative on the residents' committee. She made two close friendships and participated in more activities than expected. Margaret and her family were very happy with the changes to her life and outlook. Through identifying possible sensory loss, making the appropriate referrals and using simple aids and devices, Margaret now looks forward to an active role in her new residential setting.

conclusion

Assessment of sensory loss is extremely important in all older people. There are many strategies that can be implemented to assist in the daily living and enjoyment of life for all people experiencing sensory loss. Ageing does not preclude the possibility of retaining existing, or improving, vision or hearing. All health care professionals can begin the processes for assessment and can determine whether further investigation is required.

study questions

1 Discuss the necessity for accurate assessment of sensory loss in older people.
2 Identify some practical strategies for assisting older people with sensory loss to maximise their remaining skills and increase their repertoire for independence.
3 Using the assessment checklist in Appendix 12.2, undertake an assessment of an older person who has vision loss. Outline the advantages and disadvantages of the tool in your practice.

references

Australian Bureau of Statistics (ABS) (1993), *Disability, Ageing and Carers Survey*, ABS, Canberra.

Boothroyd, A. (1968), 'Statistical theory of the speech discrimination score', *Journal of the Acoustical Society of America*, 43, pp. 362–7.

Erber, N. P. and Osborn, R. R. (1994), 'Perception of facial cues by adults with low vision', *Journal of Vision Impairment and Blindness*, 88, pp. 171–5.

Horowitz, A., Teresi, J. and Cassels, L. (1991), 'Development of a vision screening questionnaire for older people', *Journal of Gerontological Social Work*, 17, pp. 37–56.

Kirchner, R. and Peterson, R. (1980), 'Multiple impairments among non-institutionalised blind and visually impaired persons', *Journal of Vision Impairment and Blindness*, 74, pp. 42–4.

Klein, R., Klein, B. E. K. and Lee, K. P. (1996), 'The changes in visual acuity in a population: The Beaver Dam Eye Study', *Ophthalmology*, 103, pp. 1169–78.

McArdle, P. (1997), 'Sensory impairment and mental disorders in old age', *Proceedings of the World Congress of Gerontology*, Adelaide.

MacPhee, G. J., Crowther, J. A. and McAlpine, C. H. (1988), 'A simple screening test for hearing impairment in elderly patients', *Age and Ageing*, 17, pp. 347–51.

Osborn, R. R., Erber, N. P., Rapson, W. M., Galetti, A. and Bennett, J. (2000), 'Effects of background noise on the perception of speech by sighted older adults and older adults with severe low vision', *Journal of Vision Impairment and Blindness*, 94, pp. 648–53.

Parker, W. and Osborn, R. R. (1997), 'Functional hearing assessment', *Proceedings of the World Congress of Gerontology*, Adelaide.

Reinsch, S., MacRae, P., Lachenbruch, P. and Tobis, J. (1992), 'Attempts to prevent falls and injury: A prospective community study', *The Gerontologist*, 32, pp. 450–6.

Sanchez, L., Andrews, G. and Boyd, L. (1998), 'The role of self-report in the identification of hearing loss in older Australians', *Proceedings of the Australian Association of Gerontology Conference*, Melbourne.

Schow, R. I. and Nerbonne, M. I. (1982), 'Communication screening profile: Use with elderly clients', *Ear and Hearing*, 3, pp. 135–47.

Ventry, I. M. and Weinstein, B. E. (1982), 'The hearing handicap inventory for the elderly: A new tool', *Ear and Hearing*, 3, pp. 128–34.

Voeks, S. K., Gallagher, C. M., Langer, E. H. and Drinka, P. J. (1993), 'Self reported hearing difficulty and audiometric thresholds in nursing home residents', *The Journal of Family Practice*, 36, pp. 54–8.

Ward, J. A., Lord, S. A., Williams, P. and Anstey, K. (1993), 'Hearing impairment and hearing aid use in women over 65 years of age', *The Medical Journal of Australia*, 159, pp. 382–4.

Worral, I., Hickson, L. and Dodd, B. (1993), 'Screening for communication impairment in nursing homes and hostels', *Australian Journal of Communication Disorders*, 21, pp. 53–64.

Appendix 12.1: Care planning

nursing care plan

Goals in nursing care plans need to be objectively defined. That is, they need to be measurable. The example above is an example of a goal that is difficult to measure. The goal 'to maximise hearing' is difficult to measure. Nursing notes often include comments such as 'strategies as per care plan are effective'. This is not directly measuring changes in communication behaviour with a resident. Following are suggestions on how best to assess for hearing loss and how to document findings.

There is more than one goal that is associated with a hearing loss. When possible, nursing staff should break up the goals. Goals should be objectively defined to allow accurate measurement.

hearing impairment

Goals and strategies
1   To alter the environment to optimise hearing function and communication. Strategies to achieve this:
   • reduce background noise
   • face the person
   • reduce the distance between communication partners
   • reduce glare sources (eg, close curtains)
   • direct light sources onto your face, not the resident's
   • reduce reverberation sources—more soft surfaces and less hard surfaces
   • reduce distractions.
2   The resident will use visual cues to augment comprehension of auditory information (similar to speech reading). Strategies to achieve this:
   • observe the speaker's face
   • use facial expressions or cues or other non-verbal cues
   • resident should wear eyeglasses if this assists vision
   • sit close to speaker
   • direct light source onto your face
   • avoid overhead lighting
   • identify the most effective strategies to help with visual perception
   • give the resident time to respond and to work out the context.
3   The resident and communication partner will use effective communication strategies to facilitate fluent conversations and reduce or repair communication breakdown. Strategies to achieve this:
   • slower speech rate
   • short sentences
   • clear speech
   • make sure mouth is visible

- repetition
- clarification
- rephrasing sentences
- using familiar vocabulary
- confirming that resident and partner have understood
- eliminating use of sentences or phrases that are redundant
- use of other environmental strategies
- gain full attention before speaking
- give time to respond
- use of gesture and other visual stimuli
- slightly exaggerate articulation
- use hearing aid or assistive listening device
- give context
- modify conversation if person is tired or ill.

4   The resident will use their hearing aid or assistive listening device in all appropriate environments to optimise hearing and conversational fluency. Strategies to achieve this:

- recognise perceptual difficulties
- put in hearing aid each day (or other more specific times)
- adjust volume to suit resident
- ensure maintenance of hearing aid
- use of appropriate adaptive devices (eg, induction loop, earphones for TV).

Evaluation   For this nursing care plan to be successful, nurses have to develop the necessary skills to accurately evaluate the resident's progress. They need to be trained to assess conversations quickly and uniformly to achieve this goal. The two areas relevant for this are:

- conversational fluency
- conversational effort.

Conversational fluency and effort are rated on a four point rating scale (Erber and Osborn, 1994). This evaluation can then appear on the nursing care plan. Thus, positive changes in communication will be noted. Nursing staff would also have to be familiar with *all* of the strategies mentioned previously to effectively and efficiently communicate with residents. It is important that, when nursing staff are evaluating progress, they note changes in residents' general function. This may alter the nursing diagnosis and lead to different goals and interventions.

vision impairment goals and strategies

1   To maximise the individual's awareness of people and ensure a secure and safe environment for the individual in the nursing home setting. Strategies to achieve this:

Appendix 12.1: (continued)

- introduce self when entering a room
- use touch (back of your hand to the back of their hand) to initiate communication
- tell the resident what you are doing in their room
- let the resident know when you are leaving the room.

2   To maximise the resident's use of non-verbal cues in conversation. Strategies to achieve this:

- position yourself in the best position for the resident to see you (ask resident what this is or write in the plan)
- speak a little slower and more clearly to aid processing of speech
- pause before and after key words and phrases
- reduce other visual distractions
- face the light source
- ensure your mouth is not covered
- do not chew gum, smoke etc., when talking to the resident
- use verbal acknowledgment when listening (eg, a head nod accompanied by a 'hmm' (which lets the resident know you are listening)
- reduce glare in the room.

3   To more frequently provide instructions to conversation partners about what strategies help them most with vision. A strategy to achieve this is to encourage and ask the resident to provide clear strategies that partners can use to increase visual perception.

4   To ensure that the resident's immediate living environment remains familiar and consistent. Strategies to achieve this:

- tell the resident about any changes to their room
- put things back where you find them
- use specific language to describe locations (eg, 'on the table under the lamp' rather than 'over there')
- ask the resident how they would like things arranged (eg, 'Would you like the door opened or closed?') and then let the resident know what you have done
- tell the resident where food, drink etc., is using clock face orientation (eg, 'Your meat is at 9 o'clock and your carrots are at 12 o'clock').

Appendix 12.2: Assessment checklist

Assessment of each individual with sensory loss will vary depending on information gained from prior assessments and areas identified by the individual and their family. Presented are suggestions of assessment and screening items that should be included when assessing communication and sensory loss. Referral to other professionals may be appropriate and it is recommended that this take place if necessary.

vision and communication

*   Person's known vision loss: glaucoma   yes/no
                                           macular degeneration   yes/no
                                           diabetic retinopathy   yes/no
                                           cataracts   yes/no
*   Person's self-report of communication difficulties related to vision loss:

....

....

....

oral/interpersonal communication

*   Can the person see someone entering the room?   yes/no
*   Does the person have difficulty in turn taking within groups?   yes/no
*   Can the person perceive basic lip movements?   yes/no
*   Can the person perceive basic head movements?   yes/no
*   Can the person perceive basic eye movements?   yes/no
*   Can the person copy the following movements?

                  oo ....

                  ee ....

                  ah ....

Lips   I ....

                  f ....

                  th ....

Head   shake head ....

                  nod head ....

Eyes   eyes L side ....

                  eyes R side ....

written communication

*   The person is able to read normal sized print.   yes/no
*   The person is able to read large print.   yes/no
*   The person is able to read print with magnification.   yes/no
*   The person is unable to read visually (uses talking books).   yes/no

Appendix 12.2: (continued)

- The person is able to write with normal pen and paper.   yes/no
- The person is able to write with a thick pen and lined paper.   yes/no
- The person uses templates for writing.   yes/no
- The person is able to sign using a signature template.   yes/no

hearing and communication

- Person's known hearing loss: mild   yes/no

                                        moderate   yes/no

                                        severe   yes/no

                                        profound   yes/no
- Person's self report on impact of hearing loss on communication.

....

....

- Does the person use amplification for communication?

                                        Hearing aid   yes/no

                                        Assistive listening device yes/no
- Otoscopic examination: Excessive cerumen was   yes/no

                                        present
- The person has a fluent conversation: one to one   yes/no

                                        in a group   yes/no
- Tick the following to show what the person needs in their environment for the most fluent conversation:
    - reduced/no background noise   ....
    - distance of 0.5 to 1 metre   ....
    - good focal lighting on partner   ....
    - an echo-free room   ....
- The following speech strategies improve communication:
    - Slower rate
    - Short sentences
    - Clear speech
    - Make sure mouth is visible
    - Clarification
    - Rephrase sentences
    - Gain full attention before speaking
    - Give time to respond

Other relevant information related to hearing:

....

....

assessment of elder abuse

Susan Kurrle

chapter summary

This chapter gives an overview of the issue the abuse and mistreatment of older people. It covers the definition and typology of elder abuse, the factors that contribute to abuse and identification of the different types of abuse. It describes the assessment process and provides advice on how elder abuse can be managed.

objectives

After reading and reflecting on this chapter, you will be able to:

- understand the concept and definition of elder abuse
- understand the factors that contribute to the occurrence of elder abuse
- identify the various types of abuse
- assess individual cases of abuse
- implement the most appropriate options for intervention in cases of elder abuse.

acknowledgment

The content of this chapter draws heavily on the author's previous publications and presentations, particularly the handbook by the author and Paul Sadler, *Assessing and Managing Abuse of Older People.*

introduction

Abuse and mistreatment of older people, or elder abuse as it is usually known, is not a new phenomenon but until recently it has gone largely unrecognised in Australia. Only over the last ten years has the issue of abuse achieved professional and public prominence, and research throughout Australia has confirmed the significance of abuse as a social, medical and legal problem in the Australian community.

Over the past 20 years, the issue has been researched widely in North America where it has been addressed through a range of measures, including the development of adult protective services and the introduction of mandatory reporting of elder abuse in most states in the USA. In Australia, action has occurred at both Commonwealth and state government levels, initially with the formation of task forces and working parties to look at ways of dealing with elder abuse. As a result of recommendations from these groups, states have developed specific policies on elder abuse and education programs have been undertaken. Many agencies dealing with older people now have protocols in place for management of elder abuse. Mandatory reporting has not been recommended as appropriate at this time.

This chapter provides advice to nursing professionals about how to recognise, assess and manage cases of elder abuse. It looks at the ethical dilemmas that may arise in management, and draws on past and current research to provide some framework for dealing with this complex problem.

barriers to the detection of abuse

There are still many barriers to the detection of abuse, which result in it remaining a hidden or under-reported problem.

- There is still both professional and public unawareness of the problem.
- Victims of abuse are often unable to report the abuse. They may be socially isolated and hidden from outside scrutiny when abuse occurs in the home, or they may be unable to communicate adequately because of dementia, speech problems or language barriers.
- Victims are often unwilling to report abuse. They are ashamed to admit that abuse is occurring at the hands of close family members,

perhaps a spouse or an adult child. They fear retaliation from the abuser, and most importantly, they fear removal from their home and subsequent institutionalisation.

- The symptoms and signs of abuse may easily be attributed to age-related changes or disease.
- Older people may not seek out help because they are unaware of their rights, or may believe that legal (or other) interventions are ineffective.
- Societal attitudes, including the negative stereotyping of the older person as non-productive, may lead to lack of recognition of the problem.
- There is often a reluctance in the community to report suspected abuse because of concern about confidentiality, or interfering in a family matter, or a fear of being legally involved.

definition of elder abuse

Elder abuse is any pattern of behaviour that causes physical, psychological or financial harm to an older person. The abuse occurs in the context of a relationship between the abused person and the abuser, and this therefore excludes self-mistreatment and self-neglect from the definition. The abuser may be a family member, friend, neighbour, paid carer or other person in close contact with the victim. Crime or assault in the street or at home by strangers, and discrimination in the provision of goods services, are specifically excluded in this definition. Most often the abuse we are describing will occur in relation to people aged 65 years or older. However, it is acknowledged that abuse of vulnerable adults occurs in all age groups, and a 45-year-old person with multiple sclerosis may be as much at risk of abuse as an 80-year-old with Parkinson's disease. Anyone with a chronic disability may be at increased risk of abuse.

types of abuse

There are different categories of abuse, and it is important to identify the specific type of abuse as there are different contributory factors and interventions for each type.

- Physical abuse: the infliction of physical pain or injury, or physical coercion. Examples include any form of assault such as hitting, slapping, pushing or burning. It includes sexual assault and physical restraint.

- Psychological abuse: the infliction of mental anguish, involving actions that cause fear of violence, isolation or deprivation, and feelings of shame, indignity and powerlessness. Examples include verbal intimidation, humiliation and harassment, shouting, threats of physical harm or institutionalisation, and withholding of affection.
- Financial or material abuse: the illegal or improper use of the older person's property or finances. This would include misappropriation of money, valuables or property, forced changes to a will or other legal document, and denial of the right of access to, or control over, personal funds.
- Neglect: the failure of a care giver to provide the necessities of life to an older person (ie, adequate food, shelter, clothing, medical care or dental care). Neglect may involve the refusal to permit other people to provide appropriate care. Examples include abandonment, non-provision of food, clothing or shelter, inappropriate use of medication, and poor hygiene or personal care.

factors contributing to the occurrence of abuse

No one factor can explain the complex issue of abuse, and a number of theories have been put forward. Most researchers acknowledge that a combination of these categories of abuse is often involved in the occurrence of individual cases of abuse. It is very important that these contributory factors are examined in the context of a population where an increasing proportion are elderly and there is an increasing prevalence of age-related diseases such as dementia. Government policies are advocating community care, and in light of the limited resources available, are possibly placing extra strain on family carers. The factors that contribute to abuse include increased dependency of the older person, abuser psychopathology, family dynamics and carer stress.

increased dependency of the older person

Older people are more vulnerable to abuse when they are helpless or dependent on others for assistance. This dependency may be because of physical impairments such as Parkinson's disease or stroke, or cognitive impairments such as dementia. In the majority of neglect cases, dependency is the primary contributory factor.

abuser psychopathology

The personality characteristics of the abuser are a major factor in the mistreatment of older people. Alcoholism, drug abuse, psychiatric illness and cognitive impairment in the abuser are highly significant as contributory factors in cases of abuse. In many cases of physical and psychological abuse, abuser psychopathology is implicated as the major contributory factor.

In cases of carer abuse, where carers are abused by the people for whom they are caring, dementia or psychiatric illness is frequently present in the abuser. A large number of carers of people with dementia experience aggression from the person for whom they are caring at some stage in the illness.

family dynamics

In some families, violence is considered the normal reaction to stress, and it may continue from generation to generation. In some cases, the abuser was abused as a child by the person they are now abusing. Marital conflict resulting in spouse abuse can continue into old age, and in many cases of elder abuse there has been a long past history of domestic violence. When two or more generations live together, intergenerational conflict can occur because of different values and expectations.

carer stress

The responsibility for providing physical, emotional and financial support to a dependent older family member can generate great stress. Financial difficulties, inadequate support and lack of recognition for the caring role, and personal stress, can all contribute to this stress. In many cases, other contributory factors are already present and this additional stress on the carer appears to be the factor that triggers the abuse.

the extent of the problem

The extent of abuse of older people has been difficult to estimate because of marked under-reporting of the problem, the difficulty of researching such a sensitive topic, and the varying definitions of abuse that have been adopted. However, reliable population-based studies in the USA, Britain and Canada have shown that between 3 per cent and 5 per cent of the elderly population living in their own homes are victims of abuse.

No similar community-based sample figures are available in Australia. However, several research studies looking at older people referred to aged care services in both rural and urban Australia have shown that over a one-year period, between 3 per cent and 5 per cent of clients living at home were victims of abuse.

the abuser

The majority of abusers (80 per cent to 90 per cent) are close family members, either the victim's spouse, adult child or other close relative, and they usually live with the victim. They may be financially dependent on the person they are abusing. Research suggests that spouses tend to be involved more in physical abuse and children in financial abuse. Australian and overseas studies show that approximately half the abusers will have significant problems of their own, including physical and mental health problems.

Although poor financial circumstances, poverty and lack of resources may play a part in the occurrence of abuse, it is seen in all socioeconomic groups, in urban and rural settings, and in all religious and racial groups.

identification and assessment of abuse

One of the major problems in dealing with abuse is the difficulty in recognising it. It is necessary to be on the alert because symptoms and signs of abuse are often subtle, and are attributed to the ageing process because the person is old and frail. Older people may be reluctant to admit that they are being abused by a family member or care giver on whom they rely for their basic needs.

symptoms and signs of abuse

It is important to remember that the presence of one or more of the signs listed below does not necessarily establish that abuse is occurring, as many of these are seen in frail older people with chronic disease. Ageing skin may bruise more readily, bones may fracture more easily due to osteoporosis, and falls may occur more often due to degenerative changes or disease in the central nervous system. It should also be noted that the severity of abuse can vary substantially. In some cases one incident may constitute abuse (eg, theft or physical assault), in other cases one incident may not be abusive (eg, the case of a stressed carer shouting once at a relative with dementia). However, the presence of any of the signs listed below should alert one to the possibility of abuse.

physical and sexual abuse

This type of abuse includes punching, kicking, beating, biting, burning, pushing, dragging, scratching, shaking, arm twisting, sexual assault and any other physical harm to an older person. It includes physical restraint such as being tied to a bed or chair, or being locked in a room.

- Look for a history of unexplained accidents or injuries. Has the older person been to several different doctors or hospitals? It is important to check on conflicting stories from older person and care giver, and on discrepancies between the injury and the history. There may have been a long delay between the injury occurring, and reporting for treatment.

- Any story of an elderly person being accident prone should be viewed with suspicion, as should multiple injuries, especially at different stages of healing, and untreated old injuries.

- Medical and nursing staff should undertake a good physical examination where possible. However, in the absence of a formal physical examination, other practitioners can note the presence of bruising and abrasions on exposed areas such as the face, neck, forearms and lower legs.

- On the head, look for bald patches, and signs of bruising on the scalp. This may be indicative of hair pulling.

- Watch for black eyes and bleeding in the white part of the eye. Look at the nose and lips for swelling, bruising, lacerations and missing teeth. Fractures of the skull, nose and facial bones should always alert one to the possibility of abuse.

- On the arms, look for bruising, especially bruises of an unusual shape. Consider belt buckles, walking sticks, hair brushes or ropes as instruments of injury. Look for pinch marks and grip marks on the upper arms. Victims of abuse are sometimes shaken. Look for bite marks or scratches.

- Look for burns from cigarettes, or chemical burns from caustic substances. Glove or stocking distribution of burns suggest immersion in hot or boiling water.

- Look for rope or chain burns, or other signs of physical restraint, especially on the wrists or around the waist. Older people may be tied to a bed, to a chair, even to a toilet.

- On the trunk, look for bruises, abrasions and cigarette burns. Ribs may be fractured if the victim is pushed or shoved against an object or piece of furniture.

- Medical or nursing staff should examine the genital area for bruising, bleeding, and painful areas. Check for torn, stained or bloodstained underwear. Look for evidence of sexually transmitted disease. Watch for difficulty with walking or sitting. Any of these signs may be indicative of sexual abuse.
- On the lower limbs, look for bruising, rope burns, abrasions, lacerations, or evidence of past or present fractures.

psychological abuse

This is said to have occurred when an older person suffers mental anguish as a result of being shouted at, threatened, humiliated, emotionally isolated by withdrawal of affection, or emotionally blackmailed. Psychological abuse is usually characterised by a pattern of behaviour repeated over time and intended to maintain a hold of fear over the older person.

- The older person may be huddled when sitting, and nervous with the abusive family member or care giver nearby.
- Insomnia, sleep deprivation and loss of interest in self or the environment may occur.
- Look for fearfulness, helplessness, hopelessness, passivity, apathy, resignation and withdrawal. Look for paranoid behaviour or confusion. Look for anger, agitation, or anxiety. Many of these signs may be attributed to psychiatric disorders.
- Watch how the older person behaves when the care giver enters or leaves the room. There may be ambivalence towards a family member or care giver. Often there is reluctance to talk openly, and the older person avoids facial or eye contact with both practitioner and care giver.

financial abuse

This is the improper use of an older person's money, property, or assets, by someone else. This may be more easily detected when older people are visited in their own homes.

- There may be loss of money, ranging from removal of cash from a wallet to the cashing of cheques for large amounts of money.
- Sudden or unexplained withdrawal of money from a bank account may occur.
- There may be a sudden inability to pay bills or buy food.
- Bank books, credit cards and cheque books may be 'lost'.

- There may be a loss of jewellery, silverware, paintings or even furniture.
- An unprecedented transfer of money or property to another person may have occurred.
- A new will may have been made in favour of a new friend or another family member. Power of attorney may have been obtained improperly from an older person who is not mentally competent.

neglect

This is where an older person is deprived by the care giver of the necessities of life.

- If food or drink are being withheld, there is malnourishment, weight loss, wasting and dehydration, all without an illness-related cause. The older person may have constipation or faecal impaction.
- There may be evidence of inadequate or inappropriate use of medication; for instance, the older person may be over-sedated in the middle of the day.
- There may be evidence of unmet physical needs such as decaying teeth or overgrown nails.
- The older person may be lacking necessary aids such as spectacles, dentures, hearing aids or walking frame.
- There may be poor hygiene or inadequate skin care. The older person may be very dirty, smell strongly of urine or be infested with lice. There may be a urine rash with excoriation and chafing.
- Clothing may be dirty and in poor repair, it may be inappropriate for the weather or for the person's gender.
- In some cases where the older person is immobile, they may develop pressure areas over the sacrum, hips, heels or elbows. Sometimes medical care and attention are withheld until the older person is almost moribund.

behavioural signs in the abuser

There are many behavioural signs that may be exhibited by a person inflicting abuse.

- The abuser may not want the victim to be interviewed on their own.
- The abuser may have sought medical care from a variety of medical practitioners or hospitals, or alternatively, may have refused treatment or care for the victim.

- The abuser may appear excessively concerned about the victim, or alternatively, may be unconcerned about quite severe injuries.
- The abuser may use harassment or threats of legal action towards health care professionals involved in the victim's care.

the assessment process

There are a number of points that require attention in the assessment process. In summary, these are as follows:

- Practitioners should remember that the older person has the right, assuming they are competent to do so, to refuse to answer particular questions and to decline to allow a comprehensive examination.
- It is essential to interview the suspected victim alone. Privacy is important, as older people may be reluctant to admit to the occurrence of abuse in front of others.
- The assessment interview should not be hurried and it may take some time to establish a relationship of trust where previously hidden concerns can be voiced by the victim. Questions concerning the specific incidents of abuse must be approached with tact and sensitivity.
- Note-taking during the interview may be difficult. However, detailed and accurate documentation is essential and must be done as soon as the interview is completed.
- The suspected abuser should be interviewed in as non-judgmental and non-threatening a manner as possible. Some assessment of their mental capacity and level of independence should be made. Their willingness to acknowledge the abuse and to accept assistance should be ascertained.
- A full physical examination should be performed in cases of suspected physical or sexual abuse, or neglect. This should be carried out by experienced nursing staff or an experienced medical practitioner. The presence of any indicators of abuse should be meticulously documented.
- The cognitive status of the victim must be assessed. Formal mental state testing can be performed using tools such as the Mini Mental State Examination (Folstein, Folstein and McHugh, 1975). It is essential to know the mental capacity of the victim when evaluating the information they have given, and when involving them in future decision making.

- The functional status of the victim can be documented using an assessment of activities of daily living scale such as the Barthel Index (Collin, 1990). It is also important to know the victim's living arrangements, social support system and financial status, when arranging interventions.
- An interview with the referral source is essential and contact with other informants who have information about the abusive situation is invaluable. The carer and other family members and friends must be spoken with.

It is important to take a non-judgmental approach in cases of abuse, and in many cases it may be more appropriate to look at the situation as one in which there are two victims, rather than a victim and an abuser. Attention must be paid to resolving the unmet needs of both victim and abuser, rather than simply identifying abuse and punishing the guilty party. Where there is only a suspicion of abuse occurring rather than definite proof, it is particularly important to be cautious in apportioning blame.

It is generally suggested that a multidisciplinary team, usually from a geriatric health service or aged care assessment team (ACAT), should be involved in both the assessment of cases of abuse, and intervention. These teams have extensive contacts with other services and are well placed to receive referrals, assess and manage cases, and make referrals when necessary. Appointment of a case manager is essential to oversee interventions, to provide ongoing support and to review the situation at regular intervals.

management and interventions

Understanding the dynamics of each individual abusive situation is essential so that interventions can be designed accordingly. Different types of abuse arise for different reasons. Physical abuse often relates to the personality characteristics of the abuser, and therefore intervention strategies may need to focus on the abuser rather than the victim. Situations of reverse or carer abuse, and carer stress, also commonly result in physical abuse. Neglect is often seen in cases where there is a high level of dependency of the older person due to physical or cognitive impairment, and in these cases intervention is aimed at providing assistance with the older person's care. Psychological abuse is commonly associated with a long-term history of a poor relationship between victim and abuser, and counselling may be the most appropriate response in this situation. Financial abuse may require a different approach to assessment, with a greater role for legal processes. Assessment of a person's mental capacity is important to determine which form of legal assistance or intervention is most appropriate.

ethical considerations

Each situation of abuse encountered is unique and must be considered individually. It is useful to refer to the principles of beneficence and autonomy when making decisions about intervention. Beneficence is the principle of acting in a manner that will do good and remove or prevent harm. This encompasses a practitioner's duty of care. Autonomy is the principle of self-determination. The rights of others to make their own decisions must be respected. Choice and independence, informed consent, privacy and confidentiality form part of this principle. Ideally, both these principles should be satisfied when deciding on a course of action.

Ethical dilemmas occur where there are tensions between beneficence and autonomy, such as the case of the victim wishing to stay in an abusive situation. In this case, practitioners need to balance the right of the older person to refuse any assistance with the practitioner's duty of care. Confidentiality should be respected in accordance with agency and professional guidelines; however, in a few urgent cases, the practitioner's duty of care will necessitate the contacting of police or other services, irrespective of the person's wishes.

It is very important to involve victims of abuse in decisions about their care. Individuals need to be encouraged and helped to make their own decisions, and to be given information about services they can use, and the various options available to them. Older people are capable of making decisions for themselves unless severely impaired by dementia or other psychiatric illness, and practitioners must respect that right, even though they may disagree with their decision. Where it appears that an older person lacks the capacity to make informed decisions, then assessment of mental competence is essential.

options for intervention

Ideally, intervention in cases of elder abuse seeks to achieve freedom, safety, least disruption of lifestyle, and the least restrictive care alternatives. Intervention strategies used commonly in the management of abusive situations include crisis care, provision of community support, provision of respite, counselling, treatment of the abuser, alternative accommodation and legal interventions.

crisis care

This might involve admission to an acute hospital bed, or perhaps urgent respite care in a nursing home or hostel, depending on the needs of the victim. In cases of severe physical abuse, the victim often needs to be immediately separated from the abuser.

provision of community support

The full range of community services such as home nursing, housekeeping help, continence advice, community options or linkages programs, and meals on wheels can be used to alleviate situations where abuse is occurring. Assistance with shopping and transport is of practical help to the carer. Case management is often required because of the complexity of the situation and the likelihood that multiple services will be involved. The key worker may be a community nurse, an ACAT staff member, or another health care worker. They will be responsible for the coordination of services provided to the older person.

provision of respite

This may be in-home respite, day centre respite or institutional respite. This is particularly helpful where carer stress is a problem, and where there has been a situation of neglect. If the victim is quite dependent, then often nursing home care is the only alternative.

counselling

This is an important means of intervention and may involve individual counselling or family therapy. The aim is to help the victim cope with their situation, and assist them to find a way to be safe from their abuser. It is also important that the victim be given assistance to recover from the impact of the abuse. Group therapy such as carer support groups may be useful in some situations. In cases where domestic violence is the main cause of abuse, a referral may need to be made to the appropriate services for victims of domestic violence.

treatment of the abuser

It is important to acknowledge the needs of the abuser. In cases where abuser psychopathology is a major causative factor, admission to hospital may be necessary to address the psychiatric illness or drug or alcohol problems. Psychological counselling which allows the abuser to talk openly about their behaviour may be beneficial.

alternative accommodation

Alternative accommodation on a permanent basis may be necessary. Realistically, this usually means institutionalisation, often nursing home placement, for the victim of abuse. However, in some situations where carer abuse has occurred, it is the abuser who requires nursing home placement.

legal interventions

These are hopefully a last resort, but may be the first line of intervention where criminal charges need to be laid in cases of financial abuse or severe physical abuse (particularly where there is a history of domestic violence). Older people who are competent to make their own decisions can, with support if necessary, access mainstream legal services, for instance to revoke a power of attorney or evict an unwelcome person from their home. Chamber magistrates or the police may need to be involved if an apprehended violence order or restraining order is sought. Applications to a guardianship board or tribunal can be made where victims are unable to make a decision for themselves. Guardianship boards or tribunals provide substitute decision-making functions for people who are unable to make decisions because of a disability. This disability may be a dementing illness, head injury, psychiatric illness, or physical or intellectual disability. Guardianship boards can be accessed by any individuals or service providers who have a genuine concern for the welfare of the person with a disability.

debriefing for practitioners

Dealing with cases of suspected abuse or neglect can be very demanding on practitioners, resulting in stress similar to dealing with other traumatic incidents such as sudden deaths or natural disasters. Nurses often work alone or in isolated situations, and it is important that appropriate support and supervision is offered. Debriefing should usually occur within 24–48 hours of any practitioners being involved in a traumatic event, and should be offered at the completion of each case.

use of protocols

Most agencies that have contact with older people have been encouraged to develop their own individual policies and protocols for dealing with elder abuse. These protocols should guide practitioners through the elements of identification, assessment and management and cover the areas of allocation of responsibility, duty of care, confidentiality and legal issues. Sample protocols are available from the relevant state departments or from several of the references in the reference section of this chapter (Kurrle and Sadler, 1994; NSW Ageing and Disability Department, 1996).

conclusion

Nurses are ideally placed to detect and respond to elder abuse, whether in the community or in hospital-based services such as the emergency department. As the numbers of dependent older people in the community increase, we can expect to see more cases of abuse and knowledge of the risk factors and the ability to recognise cases of abuse are important in ensuring that this hidden problem is identified and dealt with.

case studies

case 1: Mrs B

Mrs B is a 78-year-old woman who was referred to the local aged care assessment team because she had been wandering in to her neighbour's house at inappropriate times to ask for items of food. She was found to have dementia and services were arranged for her, to assist her with housekeeping, shopping and cooking. Her only family lived in another state and seemed unconcerned about her gradual deterioration. However, several months after the ACAT visit, her grandson moved in with her, ostensibly to assist in her care. All services were cancelled by the grandson.

Three months later, a request for review was made to the ACAT by the neighbour. He was concerned that Mrs B seemed to have lost weight and was quite often dressed in light clothes even in very cold weather. The ACAT nurse visited and found Mrs B lying in a filthy bed where she had obviously been incontinent on many occasions. She appeared to have lost a considerable amount of weight. The grandson was away and the only food in the house was several packets of sweet biscuits. The nurse arranged immediate admission to hospital, where a urinary tract infection, dehydration and poor nutrition were treated.

The grandson did not visit the hospital until a family conference was organised. When the suggestion of more community services was made, he insisted that his grandmother had no money to pay for any services.

As it was understood that previously Mrs B had been a woman of considerable means, an application was made to the Guardianship Tribunal for financial management, and also for guardianship. It transpired that the grandson had organised a power of attorney for his grandmother, and had moved a large amount of money into other accounts for his own use. With the making of guardianship and financial management orders, much of the money was retrieved, the grandson was removed, and Mrs B was able to afford a live-in carer.

case 2: Mr and Mrs J

Mr and Mrs J had been married for 45 years when Mr J developed Parkinson's disease. Despite Mrs J's general poor health and increasing frailty, she continued to provide all care for her husband. He refused to allow the home nursing service to assist in showering him until his wife fell in the shower and broke her wrist. When the visiting nurse attempted to shower him, he grabbed at her breasts and made suggestive comments. A male nurse took over care and no further comments were made.

Once his wife's wrist fracture was healed, Mr J insisted that his wife shower him. The male nurse continued to visit to supervise medication and noted that Mrs J often had bruising on her face. She explained that she had hit her head on the door during the night, or had fallen against a piece of furniture. Eventually, she admitted that her husband got angry with her and occasionally hit her. She felt that it was her fault as she must have provoked him. The nurse spoke with the Js' general practitioner who visited and examined Mrs J. He noted bruising of different ages on her face, trunk and arms.

A referral was made to the aged care assessment team, who arranged regular in-home respite for Mrs J, as well as assistance with showering for Mr J. Mrs J underwent considerable counselling to help her to deal with the culmination of many years of low grade domestic violence. Eventually, Mr J required nursing home placement. Mrs J's health improved markedly and she became very involved in a local handcraft group.

study questions

1 Give several reasons why elder abuse has remained a hidden problem in our community.
2 Identify the types of abuse described in Case 1, and give the likely reasons for their occurrence.

3 Discuss the ethical issues involved in Case 2, with particular reference to the principles of autonomy and beneficence.

references

Collin, C. (1990), 'More on the Barthel Index', *American Journal of Occupational Therapy*, 44 (9), p. 857.

Decalmer, P. and Glendenning, F. (1993), *The Mistreatment of Elderly People*, Sage Publications, Newbury Park, CA.

Folstein, M., Folstein, S. and McHugh, P. R. (1975), 'Mini mental state: A practical method for grading the cognitive states of patients for the clinician', *Journal of Psychiatric Research*, Nov 12 (3), pp. 189–98.

Kurrle, S. and Sadler, P. (1994), *A Handbook for the Helping Professions*, Alpha Biomedical Publications, Sydney.

NSW Ageing and Disability Department (1995a), *Abuse of Older People: Inter-agency Protocol*, NSW Ageing and Disability Department, NSW Advisory Committee on Abuse of Older People, Sydney.

NSW Ageing and Disability Department (1995b), *Legal Issues Manual*, NSW Ageing and Disability Department, NSW Advisory Committee on Abuse of Older People, Sydney.

NSW Ageing and Disability Department (1996), *Dealing with Abuse of Clients and Their Carers. A Training Kit*, NSW Ageing and Disability Department, NSW Advisory Committee on Abuse of Older People, Sydney.

index

(Page numbers in italics indicate tables, diagrams and appendices.)

optical aids for 228–9
support and assistance for
   impairment 230, *239–40*, *241–2*
vomiting 156, 165

W

weight 94
   loss of 172, 173, 181

will, living *214–18*, *219–21*
women 38
   and cancer 136–7
   needs of 25–6
wounds 129–31
   assessment of 131–4, *142–3*
   types of skin tears 132–3
   management protocol for *132*
written assessment 60–1

Nursing Older People
Issues and Innovations

Edited by Rhonda Nay and Sally Garratt

Nursing Older People: Issues and Innovations focuses on the challenges that nurses raise as essential in the provision of expert and appropriate aged care. Rather than simply offering clinical information about diseases and physical functions, this book acknowledges the progress that nurses have made, and encourages the ongoing development of innovative responses to the issues and problems presented in the field.

With contributions from leading academics and specialist clinicians, this important title reflects a culmination of many years of working with, researching and teaching about elderly people. The comprehensive theoretical content is enhanced throughout by real-world vignettes.

The broad ranging contemporary topics are organised into four key sections: policy and practice issues in which casemix funding, legislation, 'transculturalism', and euthanasia are discussed; care contexts and related issues addressing community nursing, economic fundamentalism, and staffing quality in non-acute settings; specific practice issues including sexuality, restraint, medication and palliation; and professional vision and change in which continuing education, evidence based practice and action research are explored.

Nursing Older People: Issues and innovations reflects a culmination of many years of working with, researching and teaching about elderly people. As such, it is a book that addresses the needs of postgraduate and undergraduate students in gerontic nursing courses, as well as practitioners working with elderly people in any care environment. Each chapter in some way responds to and meets the unique demands of nursing and the aged.

ISBN 0-86433-139-8

Palliative Care
Explorations and Challenges

Edited by Judith Parker and Sanchia Aranda

This important book brings together a team of thoughtful and highly reputed contributors with a wealth of experience in palliative care, who bravely and sensitively confront significant aspects of this important but difficult subject.

Taking a fresh and critical look at the scope of palliative care, the book examines options for care and controversies about care. Provision of palliative care within various contexts is discussed, as is contemporary research and the implications of this research for nursing education and practice. The implications of the shift of palliative care from the hospice movement to mainstream health care are explored. The book challenges traditional ideas about terminal illness and care of the dying, and poses difficult questions about palliative care that are the subject of debate in many countries.

Palliative Care: Explorations and Challenges does not attempt to supply easy solutions but rather demonstrates the complexities that underlie sometimes simplistic and routinised practices in the provision of palliative care. It points to the gaps in knowledge where much more systematic research is required, such as management of cancer pain and of other seriously distressing symptoms. It will be an invaluable guide for all health care students, and for health professionals and policy makers who work in this domain.

ISBN 0-86433-120-7